The Age-ability Framework
for
Emergent Seniors

Age-Ability Prayer

*God grant me courage to do
what I am able to do,
wisdom not to want to do
things I am not able to do,
and Joy achieving goals
by doing
what I am able to do.*

The Age-ability Framework
for
Emergent Seniors

Contents

Forward

Age-ability is a positive developmental or purposeful Framework for Gerontology that stands apart from Geriatrics. In answer to the question: "Does old age have a purpose?", the Age-ability Framework affirmatively answers "Yes!". Aging and aged people continue to develop or 'learn' in their environments or settings. In these learning environments, aging and aged people cope with their situations, learn from their coping then adapt to secure solutions to function well in their environments.

The purpose of old age or rather the purpose of *aging and agedness* is to be old; and, to be old as age-able as is possible within aging and aged people's actual present capacities. The environments of aging and aged people are learning or developmental environments in which aging and aged people develop by *coping* with changing situations, *learning*[1] from the coping, then *adapting* for successful personal development. (This includes people with dementia.) Caregivers support aging and aged people to successfully develop by supporting their efforts to cope, learn and adapt. Ideally, aging and aged people's community and culture also support successful adaptation into agedness.

At the very heart of the Age-ability Framework is manifest authentic existential valuation of aging and aged persons progressing into aging and agedness by aging and aged people, their caregivers and their community as a whole. It is not an approach that merely 'accommodates' or provides *only social role valorization*. Age-ability applies a different approach or paradigm to aging and agedness, than more traditional and classical approaches.

While the primary theatre or arena of the formulation of the Age-ability Framework has been long term care, what is being proposed is just as important for aging and aged people in community and home settings, as well as any other aging and aged persons' settings.

The critical activities mentioned above are Behaviours of Daily Living (commonly referred to as Activities of Daily Living), that are *preferential and intimately entwined to personal identity, self-concept and self-esteem*. The significant irreversible changes in aging can render those activities maladapted, in which case those activities within their ecological context call for alternate adaptations.

---

[1] Learning is not only cognitive and conceptual, but can also be, for example, experiential or emotive.

The Age-ability Framework is:

- ✓ strength-based
- ✓ builds or constructs from assets
- ✓ personally do-able
- ✓ values-laden

The Age-ability Framework:

- ✓ does not resist aging and agedness
- ✓ is not a deficit fix it approach to aging and agedness
- ✓ does not merely accommodate aging and agedness
- ✓ embraces aging and agedness

If disruptive and harmful behaviours by aging and aged seniors are a communication, the communication is:

"I am doing the best I can, with what I have."

It is the business of those who care for aging and aged seniors to:

- ✓ assist aging and aged seniors to form or construct their lives and personal meaning anew,
- ✓ support aging and aged seniors' creating new different but valued personally doable activities or behaviours of daily living suited to their actual capacities, and
- ✓ positively supporting the enablement of those actual present capacities, allowing
- ✓ aging and aged seniors to successfully perform to their actual and present potential in their setting or environment.

All the above is true in the performance of critical activities intimately connected the person's self-concept, identity and self-esteeming. These include communicating, ambulating, feeding, toileting, grooming, inhibiting impulses and attain self-control or self-management, and testing reality[2], etc. Significant changes to these critical life skills in aging and aged seniors are mal-adapted; the results are catastrophic for the seniors, their families and care givers.

The Age-ability Framework involves an ecological approach to human development that normalizes aging and aged-ness as a valued stage of human development into which people should successfully adapt.

The notion that all behaviour has meaning is poorly construed. *While there is a reason for each and every behaviour, not every behaviour is meaningful.* It is better that assessments ascertain

---

[2] As personal reality itself (i.e. the person in in the person's setting or environment) changes so do the tests for reality change.

the reason or causes of behaviours, as well assessments should also determine whether a behaviour is intentional or whether it has any meaning to the aging or aged person.

Age-ability frames aging and agedness based on valid assessment of capacities that are effectively enabled so that seniors successfully perform their aging and aged occupation, including personally critical occupying activities of aging and agedness.

Within Age-ability it is ok to be aging and aged. It is

- ✓ good
- ✓ right, and
- ✓ perfect

for aging and aged seniors. This is true when irreversible changes in age commence and remains true with changes in extreme aging and agedness. It is a positive stage of human development that brings its own existential merit.

Aging and aged people experience changes in critical life skills[3]. The changes in critical life skills affect aging and aged people's critical functional capacities and abilities to meet needs they were accustomed to meet successfully. In response aging and aged people are driven for better or worse, to meet their needs with solutions that are well adapted and successful or maladapted and disruptive or harmful to themselves and/or to others. Well adapted solutions to meeting the challenges of changes in critical life skills during aging and agedness are normative and natural development into aging and agedness.

Failure to successfully adapt is a root cause of behaviours that are disruptive or harmful to the senior or to others in their settings. Identified disruptive and dysfunctional behaviours[4] are indicators of failure to successfully adapt. While needed, it is insufficient to merely contain, control and maintain unmet needs or disruptive and harmful responses to unmet needs. The disruptive or dysfunction solution needs to be deconstructed and replaced with the construction or reworking of functional and successful adaptation. Aging and aged people, along with caregivers where involved should construct solutions utilizing action plans that allow for successful adaptation. The latter should engage and involve the aging and aged people to be as self-reliant and independent as possible to maximize personal self-actualization.

The Age-ability Framework identifies critical activities necessary for aging and aged people to development and sustaining their purposeful self-concept, identity and self-esteeming. These critical and necessary activities are distinct from desirable but not necessary activities that are meaningful because they are pleasurable and satisfying in the moment.

---

3 Critical life skills are discussed below and are also identified as critical life skills, Critical Occupying Activities, and behaviours or activities of daily living (BDLs or ADLs). These are not 'token' activities meant to 'fill in' or engage aging and aged people with personally meaningful but not developmentally activities necessary for personal functioning.
4 Including responsive behaviors

Age-ability prefers use of Occupational (Age-ability) Therapy using a developmental adaptive approach. What Maria Montessori, as a scientist and experimenter did with children's learning and developing in their learning or developmental environments, adaptive OT can do for aging and aged people in their learning or developmental environments. For example in Long Term Care their learning and development environments are bedrooms, dining rooms, halls, shower rooms, bathrooms and hallways. With each significant change in personal functional capacity of critical life skills, comes change in the functional capacity of the person-in-their-environment. Similarity, changes in the environment that impact on functionality, may require adapting personal functional capacity. Similar settings are in the home. Adult Day Programs and Seniors' Centres, as well as Activation Program spaces are included. Aging and aged people have an innate urge to find preferred physical, intellectual, emotional and spiritual solutions and resolutions to challenges of irreversible changes in old age. Their preference is not random but is drive by an urge to develop to meet needs and aspirations, which require successful coping, learning[5] and adapting, i.e. being good at being old. OT can answer the questions of how aging and aged seniors cope, learn, and adapt, or how they can develop and grow in their environments, then plan to remove obstacles and facilitate opportunities to enable successful developmental adaptation.

---

[5] The learning is not necessarily cognitive. It can, for example be experiential or emotive.

1. Introduction

Age-ability is an approach managing significant changes due to aging after maturity that calls for an adaptive or developmental framework. Over the years, diverse influences have come into play to shape the Age-Ability Framework approach to aging and to the aged. The work of Montessori[6], Wolfsenburger[7], Lewin[8], Bronfenbrenner[9]; Tillich[10]; experiential learning theories such as Kolb[11]; *The Activity-based Competency Development Model* with its focus on responding to change by coping, learning and adapting lifeskills; the Abilities and Asset Building movements; *The Emergent Seniors' Age-ability Framework: An Ecological Framework for Positively Supporting Changing Preferential Age-able Behaviours of Daily Living*[12]; the wide spread use of the Gentle Persuasive Approaches, the Montessori Program for Dementia and Montessori Methods for Dementia [13] in Long Term Care; as well as, the introduction of true Occupational Therapy programming into Long term Care. These influences or winds of change caught the sails of Age-ability and propelled development of the Age-ability Framework.

Work and reflection which has given rise to Age-ability as a means of framing gerontological hypotheses, notions, theories and programs relating to significant changes due to aging, was triggered by, but not limited to, the noticeable increase in 'responsive behaviours[14]' from seniors in Ontario Long Term Care homes, as well as the need to proactively resolve senior's seemingly increasing resistance to care in Long Term Care homes. Below is a sample list of salient changes in long term care in Ontario over the last 15 years or so. These changes have impacted the chemistry of change towards the positive Age-ability framing of aging and aged senior living.

---

[6] Montessori, Maria (1912). *The Montessori Method.* New York: Frederick A. Stokes Company. Montessori, Maria (1914). *Dr. Montessori's Own Handbook.* New York: Frederick A. Stokes Company. Montessori, Maria (1949). *The Absorbent Mind.* Madras: Theosophical Publishing House.

[7] Wolfensberger, W. (1972). *The Principle of Normalization in Human Services.* Toronto: National Institute on Mental Retardation.

[8] Kurt Lewin's work and formula (B=P/E).

[9] 1979. *The Ecology of Human Development: Experiments by Nature and Design.* Cambridge, MA: Harvard University Press.

[10] Existentialism of ultimate existential significance, see: Tillich, Paul. *Systematic Theology (3 volumes),* (1951–1963), University of Chicago Press.

[11] Kolb. D. A. and Fry, R. (1975) *Toward an applied theory of experiential learning.* in C. Cooper (ed.), *Theories of Group Process,* London: John Wiley.

[12] See also: Di Giovanni, Aldo. *Emergent Seniors' Age-ability Framework: An Ecological Framework for Positively Supporting Preferential Age-able Behaviours of Daily Living,* Charleston, CreateSpace , 2015.

[13] See discussion about Montessori in section 9 below.

[14] The phrase responsive behaviours has emerged in Ontario to facilitate discussion about certain behaviours associated with changes due to dementia, for example repetitive behaviours, that seem random and meaningless. By definition all behaviours have meaning of one kind or another. In effect, the definition of responsive behaviours is the same as the definition of behaviours. To keep things simple, the label 'responsive behaviours' will be set aside and the term behaviours will include what they might represent.

Ontario Long Term Care Chart of Age-ability Change Agents 2000-2015: Activation, Occupational Therapy, Social Work and Nursing Programs.				
	Activation	Occupational Therapy	Social Work	Nursing
Resident Centred Care	X		X	X
Long Term Care Act & Regulations (particularly the references to residents' rights and responsive Behaviours)	X		X	X
Best Practice Guidelines for Recreation Assessment in Ontario Long Term Care Homes	X			
ActivityPro software	X			
RAI-MDS			X	X
Residents' First	X		X	X
P.I.E.C.E.S.	X		X	X
U-First	X		X	X
Behaviour Support Ontario	X		X	X
Gentle Persuasive Approaches	X		X	X
Montessori Approach	X		X	X
Introduction of Occupation Therapy Program		X		
Broadly				
Abilities Movement				
Asset Building Movement				

These trends were also coming to the fore in community and in at-home settings.

Significant changes to activities or behaviours of daily living drives some seniors to respond to or deal with the changes by using socially disruptive behaviours. It also, causes some seniors to resist care forcing caregivers to redeploy care resources from the care itself to dealing with the resistance to care.

Seniors not in a position to 'go back' or 'restore' to their mature stage of life face the imperatives of demanding challenges requiring pressing solutions or responses. If not for all, then for many there comes a time when *the occupation of adulthood* gives way to a different *occupation in the aging and agedness*. Seniors whose capacities are significantly changed due to aging, must go forward and adapt themselves to function well in and 'occupying' all aspects of their living in *their current state*.

Functioning well begins with measuring and assessing a person's various capacities to determine the functional potential for performance. The assessment and measuring is followed by strategies and action plans to enable the capacities, as far as possible. Functioning well then happens in the performance of the enabled current capacity.

If assessment does not take into account significant irreversible changes due to aging, the assessment will be framed along lines of functionalities that no longer exist or functionalities that serve purposes other than the senior's well-being. For example, if the overall goal is to 'enable seniors to achieve maximum level of functioning *simply in order to avoid entering institutional care* such as long term care', then assessments might be directed towards attempts to shore up lost or losing capacities in order to meet the overall goal of trying to prevent changes to due to aging. The result is wasteful, maladapted and inefficient enablement strategies that undermine seniors' adapting well and experiencing well-being. Seniors and caregivers require functional capacity assessments that inform them how to live well going forward, *rather how to endure or suffer contrived losses*. The emergent senior should be encountered as an entirely new person --- even by their spouses and children. A new relationship should develop and as needed ongoing renewal of their relationship should develop.

The personal encounters of the emergent seniors significantly changing as a result of dementia can only be authentic meaningful encounters, if they are encountered as emergent, rather than with the shroud of what they were. We put the forward obstacles of yesterday's impressions that block our having present personal authentic encounters with aging and aged seniors, especially those experiencing significant change due to dementia.

In Long Term Care, Social Work supports the person's self-actualization, while Activation and Occupational Therapy work towards activating or occupying the functional capacities respectively. In terms of these two disciplines, the two together activate the personal occupation of the person.

At the same time Social Work, Nursing and Personal Support Work deal with resistance to care, socially disruptive, personally dysfunctional, as well as deleterious behaviours. Such disruptive behaviours may be the changed senior's attempts to meet needs and reach goals when the senior cannot longer meet then or reach them due to changes functional capacities as a result of natural aging. For example as when inhibition or reality testing is lost due to dementia and the person strikes their care giver during grooming.

In Long Term Care, nursing can extend nursing care further by providing (in addition to traditional restorative care to activities or behaviours of daily living), positive *adaptive-restorative* care[15], from which emerges newly formed activities and behaviours of daily living. In this nursing has a strong resource in Occupational Therapy. The same applies to the emotional, psychological and spiritual wellbeing of the resident. Nursing can use the Age-ability Framework to reframe socially and personally disruptive as well as harmful behaviours, by considering *the intentionality of the behaviour* and articulate a nursing behaviour care program that responds to that intentionality. Behaviours may be a mere reflex, for example to pain. But, they may also be maladapted behaviours that are intentionally generated by the person to deal with an issue or problem that is critical to the person. In the latter case, extinguishing or containing and controlling the behaviour does not address the underlying motivating cause. It is the maladaptation that needs to be addressed by putting an successful adaptation in place for the resident.

The Age-ability Framework as its name implies is constructed by each of the disciplines referred to above, according to *functional capacities that can be enabled and performed*, including:

- functional capacities of the person involved,
- functional capacities the person's setting, environment or eco-system, and
- dynamically dependant functional capacities of the two combined in behaviour.

---

[15] Adaptive-restorative care was first broached during 2011, in efforts to increase the effectiveness and efficiency of support care directed to changing behaviours related to maladapted activities of daily living.

The capacities are identified by way of valid assessment instruments suit to the present well-being of the senior first and foremost. Effective enablement positively enables actual present capacities. Effective enablement helps people cope with their situations, learn from their coping and helps with their adaptation so they successfully develop in their situations. Trying to enable capacities that are not present or that serve purposes other than the well-being of the present senior is ineffective, wasteful and most likely harmful.

Functional capacities are enabled using proven doable interventions and proven doable strategies or methodologies. The enabled capacities are performed according to reasonably planned expectations and goals.

Ideally the various disciplines converge by way on inter-disciplinary efforts to create a culture of Age-ability (with attendant explicit and implicit assumptions and expectations), in the persons involved, their caregivers and their communities.

In broader terms, the Age-ability Framework[16] also has useful application outside the walls of Long Term Care homes. It suits a general approach to seniors aging and the care applied to seniors aging.

---

[16] The work and efforts of many people provided the ground out of which grew ideas and concepts that were trialed and tested and revealing what work might done. The results provided stimuli to develop the Age-ability Framework. The 'team' included many people from about 2011, who should be acknowledged. Among the many involved in developing and trialing aspects of the work, the following have had notable involvement: Opi Krecouzos, Jenny Starke, Poli Pergantis, Ruel Nandwani, Juliet Nsumba, Agnes Valdez, Lula Simon, Luisa Frendo-Cumbo, Clarita Tiongson, Manuela Pechova, Luzenia Uy, Ferdinand Mulo, Sam Ho, Lisa Chan, Jingle Bisarra, Rosemary Ferraro.

2. The Positive Alternative to Deficit Thinking in Elder Care

As people age they change, just as they changed through their child development and youth development. As children and youth undergo development and emerge different as a result of their development, so seniors undergo development and emerge different as a result of their development. In the language of Occupational Therapy, each phase has an occupation which each child, youth, adult and senior should be enabled to occupy fully in turn as a child, a youth, an adult and a senior. As a naturally positive development, it is O.K. to be old, and to be getting old. In doing what old people do (rather than what younger people do); old people are doing the right thing.

It is true that some seniors naturally adapt well in response to their aging and aged conditions. In extreme aging, few seniors have had and continue to have the capacity to develop with changes capacities and to successfully adapt themselves in their environment. On the other hand, seniors who are not able to develop to significant changes in capacities and their critical life skills, are susceptible to dysfunctional and disruptive maladaptations. The number of seniors experiencing irreversible changes in critical capacities and life skills, will increase in aging. Further, each senior will experience increases in such changes as they individually age. It is also true that certain fortunate seniors develop valued aspects of themselves which in turn compensate them for the less valued changes of their aging and agedness. Those that age well are few and are counter culture. Aged champions who perform some functions even better than younger adults, are feted and celebrated for their unusual accomplishment --- but the rest their person is not equally valued as it is. Age-ability gives an appropriate value to all aspects of aging and aged seniors, including those aspects and those aging and aged seniors who are not special.

Devaluation of the emergent person is catastrophic for the individual and the community supporting the individual. The emergent person is the person to be valued as he or she is and not as he or she was. Emergent people should value themselves as they are in the present, and others should value them as the person is at present, and not as they were. This is essential for positive self-esteem, positive self-identity and positive personal functioning in daily living.

Change disturbs balance: in particular change in old age disturbs the balance of established adult living, including performance of abilities in daily living, routines of daily living, relationships, self-esteem, self-concept and identity, etc. Out of the disturbance comes brokenness that is fixed and restored; or out of the disturbance emerges a new creation that accepted and affirmed.

The Age-ability Framework is normative developmental approach to changes in old age. The Framework aspires to provide Age-able parameters, to in effect usher in 'a new age of old age'. It calls for a change in how changed aging or aged seniors see themselves and their emergence in positive vital living. It calls for change in how others (in particular caregivers) see changed seniors and their emergence into new and vital living.

It may be that aging or aged seniors undergo greater change in their aging than children do in their 'youthful' aging. If not more, then certainly more traumatic and far more mis-understood. At the time when seniors most rapidly lose their capacity to develop and adapt, they must take up significant and critical life changing developmental challenges.

In regards to aging and aged seniors, the change due to aging has been and is considered as something 'broken' or dysfunctional to be fixed by: individuals themselves; their caregivers; and, their community as a whole. Some of the efforts by aging or aged seniors to repair and restore themselves become destructive mal-adaptations.

The full weight and power of application of the medical model to health care issues encountered by aging seniors should be applied to maintain and or restore functional capacities. At the same time, such application should not turn us away from a normative development model of aging. The basis for providing what kind of care should be good assessment of aging and aged seniors capabilities, along with targeting good quality of life.

Some of the efforts to restore, mend or cure changes due to aging by care givers and communities, are deleteriously misconstrued. Efforts and attempts to help aging and aged seniors do what they do not have the capacity to do are simply destructive to seniors. Overtly or subtly encouraging them and their culture to believe that doing what they cannot do is of more value than what they can do, devalues their person.

Good assessment should determine whether a functional capacity can be meaningfully treated, restored or rehabilitated. If critical functional capacities can be meaningfully treated, restored or rehabilitated then they should be. In addition to effective application of resources to meaningfully treat, restore or rehabilitate significant reversible changes in aging and aged seniors, *the Age-ability Framework calls for realistic hope and doable aspirations in regards to self-care and in care provided by care givers. Token treatment, restoration or rehabilitation of irreversible changes in aging and aged seniors' functional capacities is a losing game that slowly disembowels aging and aged seniors while making very poor use of valuable resources.* Some of the efforts by aging or aged seniors' caregivers to repair and restore seniors to their previous state become a wasteful journey doomed to fail by way of diminishing returns and failure. Both these responses can precipitate unnecessary and harmful depression and self-loathing in aging and aged seniors.

The following chart compares: elder care framed primarily by disability, dysfunction, disease and illness, on the left; and, elder care framed to support Age-able goals that enable aging and aged seniors' present self-actualization, on the right. How the senior or the senior's caregivers frame the needs and care provided to the senior, significantly defines the senior and generates or determines the responses to the senior by the senior him or herself, as well as the caregivers' responses to the senior.

Age-unable Deficit Approach: Age-disability Framework		Age-able Positive Approach: Age-ability Framework
The aging or aged senior is defined by their dysfunction, illness, disability, sickness, etc., i.e. what they are not, or cannot do.		The aging or aged senior is defined by what he or she actual is and what he or she can actually do.
prevent and arrest, restore, rehabilitate heal, losses due to aging of capacities, abilities, enabled abilities and performance		develop and adapt, actual present capacities, enabled abilities and performance
resources allocated to deal with Age-disabled Goals		resources allocated to deal with Age-abled Goals
Ability samples	**defined by limitation focus on remedy**	**defined by actual potential focus on present actualizing**
Cognitive	loss of cognition and logic	thinks of a, b, c
Talk	impaired speech	uses sounds to communicate
Walking	poor mobility	ambulates with wheelchair
Toileting	incontinent	toilets with a brief
Navigating	wandering	explores

'The Age-ability Framework for Emergent Seniors' (AFES) is a developmental framework for supporting seniors to adapt and develop themselves in light of significant and irreversible changes due to aging. The AFES attends to the person's strengths, as they are and feeds those strengths to enable aging and aged seniors to achieve their present actual potential based on their actual capacities and functionalities. The AFES focuses especially on those changes that impact on self-concept, identity and self-esteem as a result of changes in behaviours or activities of daily living --- to the point of forming new emergent self-concepts, identities and self-esteem.

Age-able is what an aging senior can do; age-disabled is what a senior cannot do. Age-able Age-ability covers a wide field of human functioning, including physical, mental and emotional activities.

Assessment of age-able Age-ability should include perception, sensation, cognition, and responses to these in regards to behaviours or activities of daily living. And, as mentioned, in particular behaviours and activities that are intimately associated with self-concept, identity and self-esteem for it precisely these that adapt and develop as a human personality undergoes adaptation and development due to seniors' aging.

Moving forward into this time of significant change, seniors take ownership of their personal destiny in order to positively and authentically affirm themselves by proactively and fully living to their present potential.

3. The Devaluation of Aging and Agedness: a lite historical biological-medical perspective of aging and agedness

The prevailing devaluation of aging or aged seniors goes back[17] to at least to the advent of biology and the notion that human perfection is attained at human maturation when human abilities reach their potential actualization. What is socially most valued is the actualized mature person with all the potential abilities of a mature person enabled and performed productively. To this primitive understanding the human person was added biological and medical science. Out of the bio-medical model emerged the following life-line:

growth to potential maturity	mature, full abilities	decline , debilitate and disable
becoming perfect	**perfect**	**becoming and being imperfect**
activating	active	inactivating

Children are valued for their potential to mature and occupy their role as mature perfected adults. According to the bio-medical model, children can be a social benefit. They are valued. They have the intrinsic value that people should and do aspire after. Mature adults are *perfect*.

But according to the bio-medical model, seniors are… just the opposite. Seniors are 'naturally' devaluing and they are also generating a social deficit. Aging or aged seniors are the harbingers of death.

Generally the medical model approaches people as body-machines to be fixed, mended or cured in order to perform the productive activities of a mature person. For this reason, the medical model approaches seniors to arrest or reverse so called decline and debilitation, by fixing what is broken, mending what is not functioning and curing what is ailing. There is no place in the usual bio-medical model to consider aging as positive and *progressive* human development.

The notion that human perfection is human maturation fostered limiting medical and scientific theories of human development. Deviance from such 'perfection' is defective and the 'imperfecting' becomes doubly horrific when, in regards to aging it also served to also announce irreversible dying and death. Such deviants are considered disabled. Their accumulating deficit, increasing deviance and de-occupying of their mature role signals the victory of the 'disease of old age' and death of the person.

Like aging and aged seniors, the disabled (mental and physical) have historically also been devalued and their role considered a social deficit, though they were seen more as harbingers of disease, than heralds of the grim reaper as well.

Aging from a bio-medical perspective has not been considered as developmentally healthy. Old age has not been and is not included as part a healthy part of theories normal human

---

[17] It goes back a long way and it also extends out across cultures.

development. The bio-medical perspective has fostered theories of human development that mirror a bio-medical perspective. In terms of these theories, old age is a time of decline, disintegration, dying and death. This perspective has been fuelled by the perennial dear of dying that infests our 'souls', perhaps coming out of a biological drive to preserve our species.

Change in old age is to be expected and the person needs to adapt to the changes by emerging from the development with changed self-concepts, identities and self-images based on the realities of their newly acquired functionalities. Old age is rarely, if ever, approached as a stage of positive, progressive personal development, nor are developmental resources allotted to support people's positive progressive developmental adapting while aging.

Positive, progressive personal development in aging requires "a new age of old age".

4. **An Existential/Spiritual Valuating of Aging and Aged Seniors**: a new age of old age

In the long history of the bio-medical approach to what 'being human' is; there have always been some people who refused the model in favour of alternate valuations of their humanity and the humanity of others. In response to the mechanistic approach of the biological-medical model, someone(s) stand up and asserts: "I am more than my physical body!" In reality, the authentic existential significance, meaning and purpose of a purpose does not rest in the mechanics of his or her flesh and blood body.

A response from Truth beyond the material stands to say: my authentic and true person or self, which carries existential significance, meaning and purpose, is more, far more than the flesh and blood body which carries me. The biological-medical approach to fixing and repairing bodies has an important place and role in Age-ability --- it is not a defining place or role. I am defined by the existence I have: perfect in what I actually am, regardless of the conditions of body which carries me.

From the existential/spiritual perspective emerges the following life-line:

full growth to actual potential
each is perfect in his or her self
each is fully activated at each point

At each point, each existentially valued 'I', as it is --- as child… as adult… as senior---- is as valued as any other point. The person is fully alive regardless of their bodily situation; regardless of the condition of the physical and cognitive carriage that carries the person. Each point of the development line is designed to serve the person as the person actually is at that point.

As will be seen, there is a marked difference between valuing a *social role* as it is and valuing *existing itself* as it is. The former is something we individually and socially do for others. The latter is something a person does for himself or herself, based on fully enabling their actual individual capacity(ies) and performing the emergent abilities to be as much as the person can be, as they are here and now. Each aging and aged senior, as they actually are at the time, has an 'inscribed' value intrinsic to their person, which they are their caregivers should respect. This is different from an 'ascribed' social role value which given to them by others, for example their care givers or families.

Social role valorization accepts, tolerates and accommodates the role mechanically artificially assigning significance, meaning and purpose to the role. The individual passively or 'resignedly' accepts the situation, and artificially attributes artificial value to themselves based on value given by others. Personal existential valuation or valorization emerges and actively stands, in and of itself, from within the seniors actual existence and existing from which when a senior actively takes ownership of his or her existing as much as possible, as significant, meaningful and purposeful.

Existentially capacities emerge that we enable and perform or actualize. Incapacity does not emerge and we do not enable nor perform 'incapacity'.

We cannot enable a disability. In and from our actual, present existence and existing, we enable emergent abilities.

5. Existential Valuation: more than *social role* valorization

The principle of Normalization was enlarged to involve Social Role Valorization[18]. Both were and are very productive within the terms of their own parameters. Social roles can be measured and evaluated. If found to be devalued compared to other social roles, groups or communities can deploy strategies to mitigate harm or revalue the devalued social role.

Using Social Role Valorization strategies, we can *accommodate devaluated people*. Provide them with a welcomed place at the table. We can relate to them in accordance with the greater social value we place on them at the table. For example we can accommodate a person who is developmentally delayed or physically disabled and give greater currency or value to their disability or limited ability. This social valuation allotment can also apply to aging and aged seniors. We can give them a revered place and ascribe respectful honour at the table and socially value them for being old. But personally, these are not ultimately satisfying solutions.

Social role valorization attributes value in terms of social currency to the person. Our role in existence is different than our societal role. Existentially, there are other means of affirming the alternate meaning, significance and purpose of aging and aged seniors.

For seniors who have changed significantly due to aging, social role valorization from others or from themselves, is at best a consolation prize. The real prize is being accorded authentic personal existential significance, meaning and purpose.

---

[18] *A Brief Introduction to Social Role Valorization as a High-order Concept for Structuring Human Services.*
Syracuse, NY: Training Institute for Human Service Planning, Leadership and Change Agency (Syracuse University).

6. The Age-ability Liberation: a call for the development of *perfect* seniors

> *Aging and aged seniors are perfect as they are, here and now. Any imperfection they, or anyone else, might think they see in their aging and agedness, is only in the eyes of the beholder: it is not in reality itself. The Age-ability Framework is first and foremost a means of finding and celebrating the authentic value of the aging or aged individual as he or she is at the time. Following that affirmation, the aging or aged senior works within the Age-ability Framework, to exist as much as possible and as far as possible, within the realities of their actual functional capacities. Managing socially disruptive and harmful behaviours, saving the health system expense, using the available therapies, etc., are all secondary to personally celebrating aging and aged living for itself within itself even in the deep and far reaches of extreme dementia or within their extreme physical limitations.*

In our personal development, the acquisition and performance of preferred behaviours of activities (PBDLs) essential to daily living has significant and critical influence on the formation of our person, self-concept, identity and self-image. These activities or rather preferred behaviours of daily living are activating, occupying or self-actualization activities that are integral to our personal activation, occupation or self-actualization. Our response to the changes in behaviours associated with our personal identity, self-concept or self-esteem, has essential existential importance. A healthy response to such change is the formation of adapted or new PBDLs up to and including adapting into a new person.

When those functional capacities undergo significant change due to aging, the role and function of PBDLs relative to whom or what we are should progressively change or rather adapt or be formed anew as our capacities, abilities and performances of specific BDLs or of our person as a whole change. Similar adaptation or formation can be required if the dynamic functional dependence of behaviour to environment is impacted by changes in the person's environment or setting.

Seniors; abilities and the performance of their abilities should and will change when their capacity changes. In senior development, the acquisition and performance of behaviours of activities of daily living (BDLs) has significant and critical influence on the formation of their changed person, changed self-concept, changed identity and changed self-image. Mal-adaption resulting from aging (e.g. anger or frustration at not being able to control or manage urination or defection, i.e. toileting) creates significant disturbance to the individual person and others in the person's environment.

The transition or development from adult to senior has largely been approached only in terms of increasing personal and social deficits. For example when people feel a loss during the change with no sense of gain; or, when, to help keep healthcare costs down, health care systems encourage senior activation in the community only to prevent them from moving into more expense long term care sooner rather than later.

Because of the social and cultural paradigm we are in, changes in age due to dementia are generally seen by us as movement towards disability and imperfection. This generates grief and mourning on the part of care givers, friends and social associates on the one hand. At the same time it generates frustration, anger and socially disruptive behaviours on the other hand.

When the transition from adult to senior is driven by dementia, it is challenging to cast the change as positive development. We so strongly value the person's identity and self-concept, that it is difficult to let it go in order that the 'new' person can emerge and be valued as that person actually is. The challenge and difficulty is ongoing when cognitive change results in on going. Dementia is associated with loss, and consequently with grief and mourning. In reality, every loss is accompanied by an acquisition which may not be valued. We tend to not celebrate the emergent demented person's abilities, including cognitive and emotional along with the physical, as much as we endeavour to celebrate abilities that are no longer present.

Changes in seniors due to aging cast as losses, deficits or imperfection, are cast into harmful and destructive views of the person, which in turn are harmful and destructive to the person and the person's life.

Seniors should have and deserve to have an accepted and developmental paradigm for aging that allows them the ability to move towards their personal human perfection and the social valuation, they are entitled to have as significant, meaningful and purposeful aging and aged seniors.

7. Personal Paradigm Shifting[19] in Aging and Agedness

a) constructing an emerging framework or paradigm

Let's consider contextualizing the following.

What do you see? … nothing.

---

[19] Paradigm and Paradigm shifting are used here as perceptual and conceptual shifting described by Thomas Kuhn in: T. S. Kuhn, The Structure of Scientific Revolutions, 1st. ed., Chicago: Univ. of Chicago Pr., 1962. But, they are used here when the perceptual, conceptual and emotive shifting are a result of changes in the object or objects of reality triggering a need for a new frame or paradigm.

Let's turn on the light… and what we do we see? ….indifferent and meaningless splats of black ink on white paper.

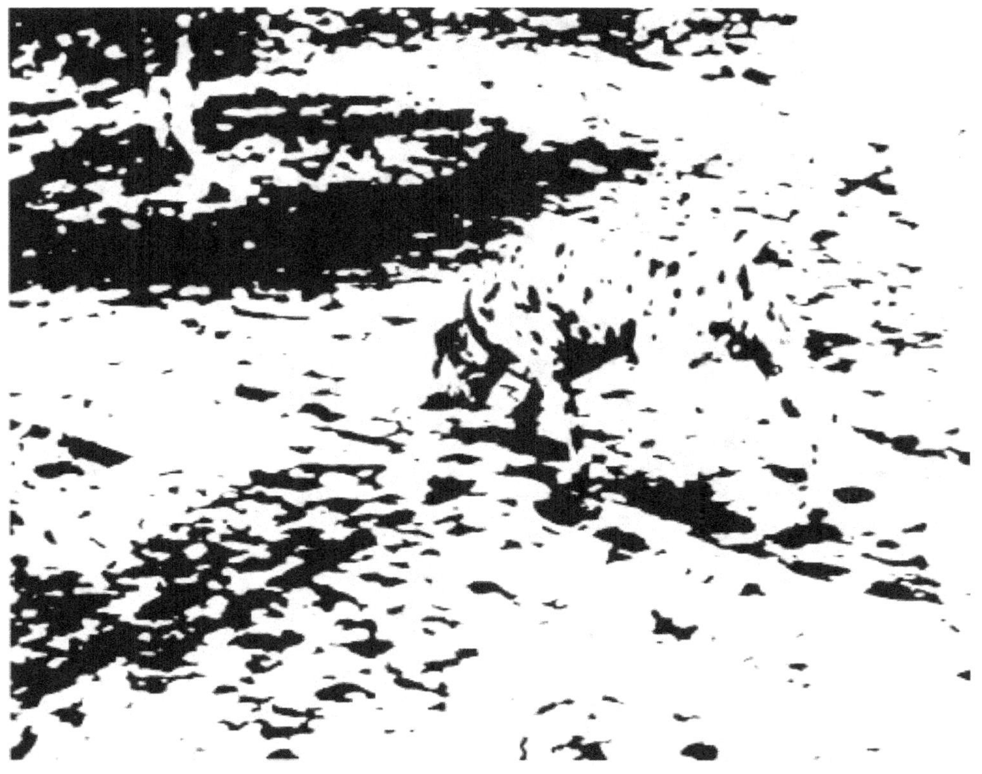

So what is in there…. Let's look again and think.   I think I see a dog

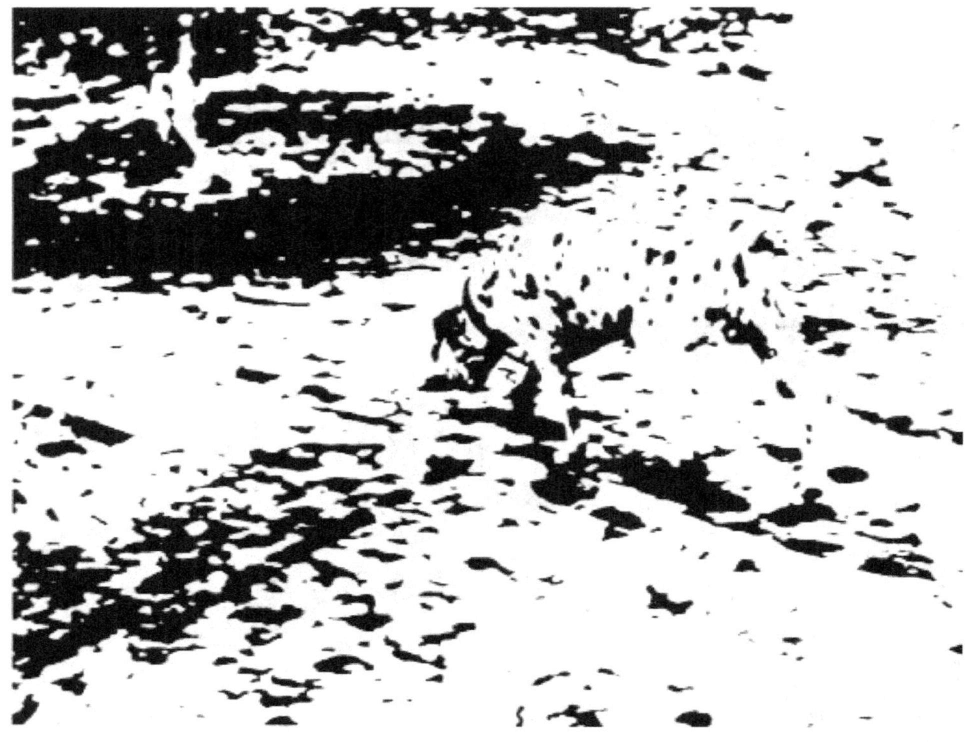

From the application of our intention, experience and values we conceive, then perceive a Dalmatian dog in the middle of the splats. Let's connect the dots and draw the Dalmatian dog. In a sense, we 'create' the Dalmatian dog.

Neat. What else is in there? Let's look again and think some more… I notice a tree, some tree shade or a garden bed, and pathways

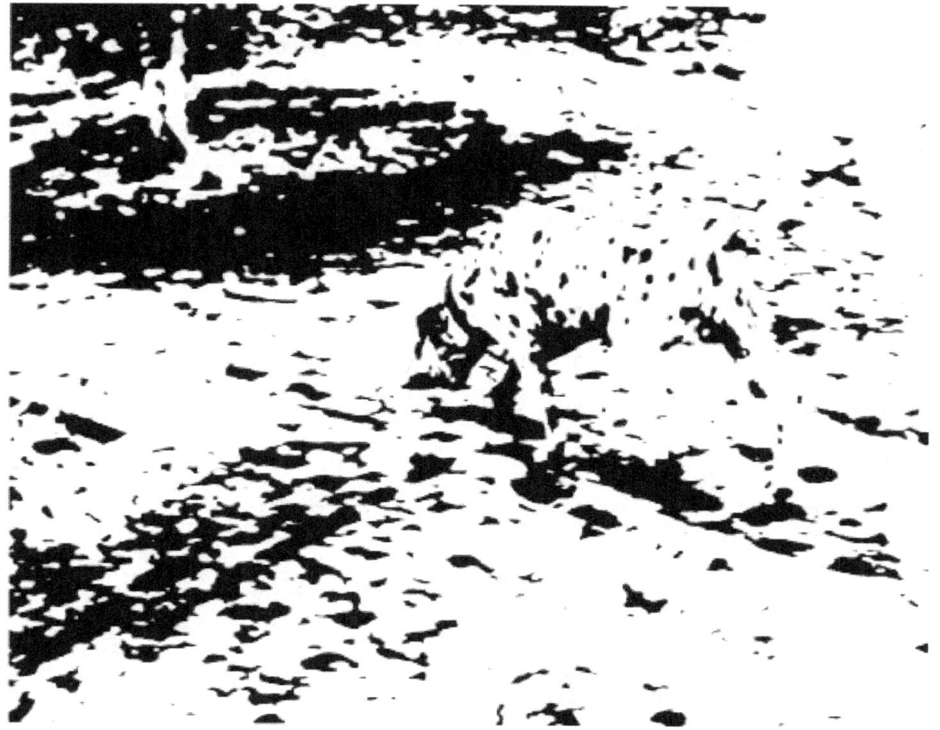

Can you see a tree in the upper right corner? a shadow at its base (or is it a garden bed); a pathway from the bottom left corner to the top right corner; and finally a path that criss-crosses the first at the page centre. Let's draw those things.

The tree base is interesting because it can go either way. Is there anything there that is not real? We create some true conceptions and some untrue conceptions; as well we create concepts of relations between what we conceive. Perhaps we also find also a woman's face underneath the dog's rear legs? The latter is not likely and is does not reflect a likely reality. We test conceptions and perceptions against 'reality' to distinguish what is true from what is not true.

We have been developing a framework by contextualizing the splats of ink using our ability to attend and focus, as well as test our perceptions and conceptualizations. We can deconstruct a framework[20]; then, using similar data or activities construct a different framework with different dynamics and different values. Such construction is like the construction of a 'Gestalt'.

The Age-ability framework is an alternative framework into which seniors, their caregivers and communities can transition. The transitioning will be triggered by irreversible changes to capacities. But, the direction of transition is governed by values, attention and focus.

---

[20] Such construction is like the construction of a 'Gestalt'.

b) transitioning frameworks or shifting paradigms

Contextualizing involves the forming or grasping of perceptions and conceptions. In pulling together the idea of the Dalmatian, one had to formulate its parts as well as the Dalmatian as a whole. There is interplay between the parts and the whole of the dog. But, the same thing applies to the parts and the whole in the parts themselves. Just as the whole has constituent parts, so the parts as whole in themselves have constituent parts. This segmentation allows for increasingly detailed task analyses, the results of which feed into the process of sensory, perceptual, emotive and cognitive formulation of the emerging framework. In this way, we fashion self-concepts and identities which enable self-esteeming systems.

In grasping the Dalmatian there was a forming. Below are several diagrams that illustrate formation involving transition. What image emerges below?

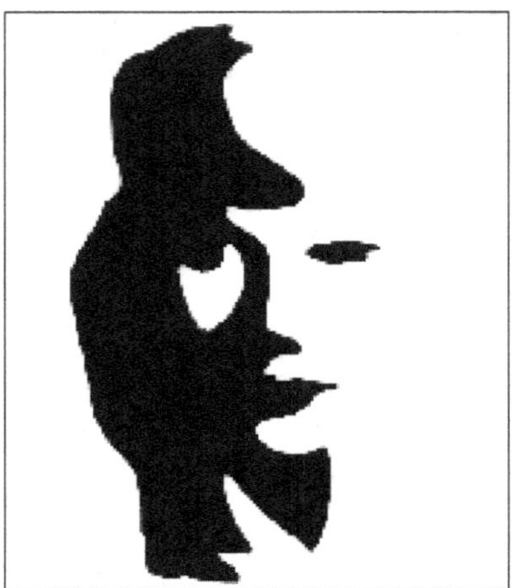

The image above can be grasped in two ways. There is an image of pretty girl and an image of a saxophone player. *Both are real images that have completely different gestalts[21]. Furthermore, we can intentionally switch or transition from image to the other.*

If this is a picture of a pretty girl then we will relate to her a certain way; and she will relate to us a certain way. Her roles and responsibilities will be formulated from her perception of herself, as well as our perceptions of her. On the other hand, if this is a picture of a fellow playing a saxophone then we will relate to the picture and its 'subject' differently, *even though the actual physical data has not changed.* The picture can be perceived or conceptualized as we choose it to be!

---

[21] The same can be said of Paradigms.

Here is another picture that can support two very separate images or subjects. Its uses and function depends on what it is perceived to be. What is the subject of the picture?

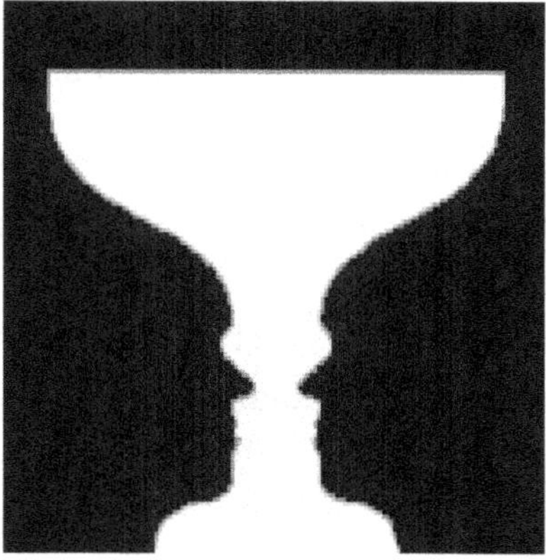

If it's a goblet then we will relate to it a certain way. Its uses and functions will be formulated from our perception of it. On the other hand, if it's two people face to face, then we will relate to the picture and its 'subjects' differently, *even though the actual physical data has not changed*. Again, based on preference we choose what the subject of the picture is to be and functionality as well as stimulus can be organized accordingly! We are the authors of what we grasp. Care givers participate in such authorship when they engage in care that involves the person as a whole.

The above 'gestalt switches' or changes are result from changes in our attention and focus. Similar, but more manifold and complex gestalt changes are at play when we consider our personal experience. The change or shift in our gestalt of images, is similar to changes or shifts in our experience of personal paradigms. In regards to ownership of work/job, the changes in gestalt are greater and more extensive than just perceptual changes. The subjects are not pictures, but living active people, who themselves have their own perceptions and conceptions of what things are and what is going on. The changes extend into roles and responsibilities, as well as uses and functions. They alter how we relate and develop. They influence identity and self-esteem. How goals and plans of action are framed is affected. How problems are framed and potential solutions to the problems is affected. The framing of the relationships between people is affected (including relationships between caregivers and the care recipients). How personal performance is measured and evaluated is affected.

The above concerns the shifting or changing of paradigms. Thomas Kuhn described the mechanics that drives **forced changes** in theoretical science paradigms[22]. Functional capacity frameworks can be cast as paradigms to explain functional capacities and inherent anomalies or various to predictable outcomes. When the working out of the anomalies or variances becomes

22 T. S. Kuhn, The Structure of Scientific Revolutions, 1st. ed., Chicago: Univ. of Chicago Pr., 1962.

intractable or exceedingly difficult, an alternate framework or paradigm might explain all the phenomena including the anomalies and variances if one can shift paradigm from one paradigm to the other. This what occurred in the field of astronomy going from a geocentric to a heliocentric solar system, moving away from Ptolemaic astronomy to the astronomy of Copernicus, Kepler and Galileo. When an existing paradigm is invested with a lot of value, the shift *is forced* by the difficulty or intractability of the anomalies or variances.

In the great expanse of astronomy, the shifting was forced observations, perceptions and conceptions that were incompatible with Ptolemaic theory. In the smaller sphere of personal functional capacities, changes in the phenomena themselves may be what creates the disruptive anomalies and variances, which in turn call for a shift in perception, observation and conceptualizing of functional capacities individually or as a whole for the entire self. If the new paradigm is maladapted, it will fail at and create dysfunction.

There are similar things at work in shifting personal paradigms from one stage of human development to the next. This applies equally well when shifting from the adult paradigm to the aging and aged paradigm.

Significant changing in functional capacities of critical life skills presents people with problems to solve in order for them to continue functioning. Kuhn illustrated the shifting of paradigmatic theories of science in his book. The same dynamic is at play in the shifting of *personal occupational paradigms*. When problems can no longer be solved or resolved within the existing personal occupational paradigm or when the resources required to deal with the problems are no longer affordable, the formation of a new personal occupational paradigm is forced. The shift in the astronomy paradigm was shift on perception and conception of the observer. What Kuhn did not consider was the need for paradigm shifting triggered by real external changes in the reality we experience. This includes changes in functional capacities or preferred behaviours of daily living that are critical life skills. In such cases the emergent alternate activities need to newly define the emergent paradigm's 'problem samples' and 'solution samples' to guide the enablement of functional capacities of the new occupation and occupational activity. With the new alternate personal paradigm comes a different but doable set of functional activities.

There a number of critical life skills that people take possession of which become core constituent parts of the person's self-concept and identity. These include Preferred Behaviours of Daily Living[23], in which the preference is driven by the integrity of the self.

In the early stages of human development the change or forming does not involve transitions of 'self'. But, as development continues, the change or forming also involves transitions of one 'self' to a changed 'self'.

---

[23] These are also referred to as Activities of Daily Living, and in terms of Occupation Therapy can be call Critical Occupying Activities.

c) shifting behaviours of daily living and preferred behaviours of daily living

Transitioning or shifting a paradigm alters our grasp of reality. In a sense for us personally it actually shifts the reality we know or conceptualize. If what changes is what reality actually is to us personally, then our relationship to the reality we conceptualize also changes. Personal paradigm shifting alters the person we conceptualize and know ourselves to be. Changes in the parts of our person that are critical, 'life and death' parts and that are at odds with the whole of our personal paradigm, will result in emotional and cognitive stresses and traumas.

In the process of human development, we go from one personal paradigm or occupation to an entirely different paradigm of occupation, which includes our physical, emotional, cognitive and even 'legal' person. We readily recognize such changes in behaviours of daily living, preferred behaviours of daily living, and we even embed accommodations for the changes in law.

We are familiar with the various stages of human development and we are familiar with and have extensive knowledge about the transitioning or shifting from one stage to another: except for the change from adulthood to aging and agedness.

In long term care, activation plans of care quickly take into account that aging and aged seniors' meaningful but not critical activities are only partially doable. The person's plans of care then calls for a *modified version of the activity*, examples include bowling or bingo playing activities. This *restorative activation* does not replace the activity. Depending on the degree of personal bonding to the activity, the aging and aged person may continue to participate one of several domains if not all. Instead of playing bingo the person participates by emotionally or intellectually watching bingo. If the bonding is intimately connected with the person's self-concept the response may not to be passive intellectual involvement, but a depression or aggression response to the loss. At some point, the person may withdraw from the bingo activity and replace the bingo activity with a different valued and meaningful activity. This transition is not merely a perceptual gestalt switch regarding the activity, but is a paradigm shifting of the person's reality and occupation.

8. Aging and Aged Seniors Adapting to Aging: Performing Actual Functional Capacities

A) Measure and assess to determine *capacity to functionally perform* physical, cognitive, emotional, social, spiritual activities.

>   Does capacity exist?
>   - If capacity exists for previous state then enable it.
>   - If capacity exists in a changed state then enable the changed capacity.
>   - If capacity does not exist then do not proceed.
>
>   When past capacity does not exist, identify a new actual functional capacity to perform.
>   - As required, determine a new suitable activity to perform based on a 'new' capacity and make plans to enable it.

B) Undertake *effective capacity enabling* (able-ing) activities (interventions) to establish the capacity as ability.

C) Undertake *performance management* of and report on enabled activities

Programs in Long Term Care That Utilize and Have Utilized Age-ability to Support Performance of Functional Capacities		
Program	Result Area	Measurement & Assessment[24]
Activation	APO Best Practice Guide ActivityPro - from program and calendar driven to person centred	ActivityPro (Functionality Assessment) Recreation/Leisure Assessment
Social Work	Behaviour Support Program (BSO)	Behaviour Assessment Tool (BAT) P.I.E.C.E.S. Assessment, MMSE, and MOCA
	Social Service Groups – Age-ability	
Peer Culture	Resident Council	
	small group	
Occupational Therapy	OT	RAI-MDS 2.0. P.E.O.
	Setting Scan	
	OT Age-ability group	
	OT Adaptive Restorative in Nursing (Feeding and ambulating)	
	OT ADL/BDL Adaptation	
Nursing	Behaviour Care	PIECES, RAI-MDS 2.0
	Adaptive Restorative – A/BDLs	RAI-MDS 2.0
	Adaptive	
Biological-Medical	Psycho-geriatric Outreach Program	
	MD Assessment	
	Nurse Assessments	RAI-MDS 2.0

---

[24] There is interdisciplinary utilization of the assessments undertaken by particular disciplines.

9. Activation: looking at a *shifting framework or paradigm*

A consideration of therapeutic recreation and occupational therapy sets a stage to view the development of activation programs and programming from an Age-ability perspective.

Definition and purpose of Therapeutic Recreation[25]

> **Therapeutic Recreation Ontario endorses the following definition:**
> Therapeutic Recreation is a process that utilizes functional intervention, education and recreation participation to enable persons with physical, cognitive, emotional and/or social limitations to acquire and/or maintain the skills, knowledge and behaviours that will allow them to enjoy their leisure optimally, function independently with the least amount of assistance and participate as fully as possible in society. Therapeutic Recreation intervention is provided by trained professionals in clinical and/or community settings.
>
> **The purpose of Therapeutic Recreation (TR)**
> The purpose of TR is to enable all individuals to achieve quality of life and optimal health through meaningful participation in recreation and leisure. The profession recognizes the importance of the recreation experience and supports all individuals in having full access to and the freedom to choose recreation and leisure opportunities.

Occupational Therapy differs in directing itself to enabling meaningful *occupations*, (including recreational activities), which occupations in effect determine the person.

Definition and purpose of Occupational Therapy[26].

> **As defined by the Canadian Association of Occupational Therapists**
> Occupational therapy is the art and science of enabling engagement in everyday living, through occupation; of enabling people to perform the occupations that foster health and well-being; and of enabling a just and inclusive society so that all people may participate to their potential in the daily occupations of life (Townsend& Polatajko, 2007, p. 372). …
>
> Occupational therapists define an occupation as much more than a chosen career. Occupation refers to everything that people do during the course of everyday life. Each of us has many occupations that are essential to our health and well-being. Occupational therapists believe that occupations describe who you are and how you feel about yourself. A child, for example, might have occupations as a student, a playmate, a dancer and a table-setter.

---

[25]© 2014 Therapeutic Recreation Ontario, https://www.trontario.org/about-therapeutic-recreation, September 2015
[26] © 2003-2015 Canadian Association of Occupational Therapists, http://www.caot.ca/default.asp?pageid=3824, September 2015.

Occupational therapy can more readily align itself with activities or preferred behaviours of daily living. The notion of occupation and its role catches certain personal behaviours or activities of daily living (PBDLs/ADLs) essentially connected to a person's self-concept, identity and self-esteem.

The development of activation has been influenced by Maria Montessori's work and ideas on human development and education. This is seen for example in the notion that activities should be designed according to the participant's actual functional capacities, given the particular setting the participant is in at the time. The focus is on what the person can actually do and enabling them to successfully perform what they can do and choose to do. While past preferences may help develop a program of activation activities for a participant, present preferences override past preferences. In addition, good activation planning anticipates future preferences and supports the participant to acquire the skills and experience to successful do what they will prefer to do. All this is managed with the notion that participants will choose to do what benefits them, not what might harm them in one way or another. As people change, they will select what works for them and so develop accordingly. Activation is a means of supporting aging and aged seniors to adjust to their changing capacities and changing environments, and activation can be usefully and productively used to that end.

Under influences from nursing care and social workers concerned with behaviours or activities of daily living, and with managing behaviour care, activation programming and programs in Ontario are evolving towards the occupational therapy frame of reference. This trend has been accelerated by the introduction of *the strong language in the Ontario Long Term Care Act and regulations in regards to residents' rights*. This language has triggered best practices that call for functional assessments and differential programming based on the enablement of aging and aged people's *actual* capacities. Giving priority to restoring or re-establishing past functionality that no longer exists, is set aside. It has also been intensified by the widespread use of strategies, such as the Gentle Persuasive Approaches, the Montessori Program for Dementia and Montessori Methods for Dementia [27] to deal with maladapted behaviours in long term care homes.

The past purpose for activation programs for seniors, for example in nursing homes, was to keep seniors active physically, emotionally, cognitively, etc. Activation programming utilized enjoyable leisure and recreational activities to engage as many seniors as possible in keeping active. Programmed activities were intended to 'put off' aging due to inactivity and prevent accelerating debilitation due to changes in old age. Activation programming was a way of keeping seniors busy and active, so that people would not wither away, as it were.

Over the last few decades, activation in long term care has been changing. Good activation programming now intentionally supports people to do what they can do creating opportunities for seniors to self-actualize by finding significance, meaning and purpose for themselves in goals they can set and accomplish. Activity staffs do not plan for or encourage seniors to do what they are not able to do, nor spend time trying to do what they cannot do. The result is that at times, seniors self-actualize by successfully attaining the goals they set for themselves. *The purpose of Activation programming in long term care is and has become to support aging and aged seniors to do well at doing what they can do.*

---

[27] See discussion about Montessori in section 9 below.

Some years ago, Activation in long term care moved towards increased individualized assessments and differential programming for residents in long term care. This trend was significantly accelerated with the advent of The Activity Professionals of Ontario's *'Best Practice Guidelines for Recreation Assessment in Ontario Long Term Care Homes* '[28], during the roll out of Ontario's 2007 Long Term Act and Regulations. In addition, the advent of Ron Martyn's *ActivityPro software*[29] at about the same time in Ontario, brought forward more focussed functional assessments in some activation programs that delved deeper into seniors' functional capacities for activation activities and tracked changes in functional capacities to shape doable individualized differential programming goals for seniors. Activation has moved closer to Maria Montessori's fuller method of intervention. These changes and tools have provided means of *better purposing Activation programming* in long term care.

In recent years, Activation has been increasingly used to help manage disruptive intentional behaviours. Activation applied its tried and effective approach of supporting seniors to focus on and to do what they can do and rather than on what they can no longer do. This was greatly helped by the increased usage of *Gentle Persuasive Approaches* (GPA) and the *Montessori Program for Dementia* as well as the *Montessori Methods for Dementia*[30] approach by both nursing and activation departments.

There were significant changes to nursing in long term care with the advent of enforcement of the Long Term Care Act (2007) and its Regulations; the introduction of RAI-MDS (Resident Assessment Instrument – Minimum Data Set); the extensive P.I.E C.E.S.[31] training for nurses but that spilled over to some activation and social work programs; and, considerable effort demanded by the roll out of the Behaviour Support Ontario Program. Activation utilizes the assessments undertaken by other disciplines in long term care in it program and individual program planning. These changes facilitated positive inter-disciplinary care involving nursing, social work and activation. Unlike therapeutic recreation goals of enabling recreation and leisure activity per se, activation in long term care is increasingly used by nursing and social services as means to their ends.

The wide spread and enthusiastic use of the Camp's *Montessori Programming for Dementia*[32] (MPD) and Elliot's *Montessori Methods for Dementia*[33] have been well received in recent years, especially in dementia care. Some approaches, like Camp's, are an "I am still here." approach. In contrast, Maria Montessori's approach can be considered am "I am going there." approach. Maria Montessori would not favour a 4 year old stating "I am still here." referring to his or her previous 3 year old self. She would not have set out to sustain the 3 year old self by way rehabilitation or restoration, nor would she be supportive of maintaining the 3 year old person, who has actually become 4 years old. Montessori's observations concluded that children displayed a natural tendency to develop. Children cope with their situations, learn from their coping then adapt. The educator's role was to remove the child's and the child's setting's obstacles and impediments to that natural development. She did make use of sensory and

---

[28] Activity Professionals of Ontario
[29] See activitypro.net website.
[30] See discussion about Montessori in section 9 below.
[31] See P.I.E.C.E.S website at: http://www.piecescanada.com/
[32] Camp, C.J. (2010), Origins of Montessori Programming for Dementia. Non-Pharmacologic Therapies in Dementia, 1(2) 163-174.
[33] Gail M. Elliot, *Montessori Methods for Dementia,* McMaster University, 2011. Elliot seems to go further along the Maria Montessori way.

experiential methods to both remove obstacles and impediments from development, and to facilitate opportunities for development. What is true for child development is equally true for aging and aged people's development.

The "I am still here." approach strives to retain the person's past occupation in light of significant changes in critical life skills. Its interventions are rehabilitative, restorative and are at least maintenance oriented. The focus on maintenance can foster a 'dynamic restraining' of aging and aged people by engaging them in and holding them with captivating sensory stimulation and past 'out of context' activities34, in order to prevent responsive disruptive or harmful behaviours. While it has its use, such dynamic restraining is not the preferred intervention.

The "I am going there." approach strives to support the person's successful coping, learning and adapting of critical life skills based on actual present functional capacities of the person in their setting or environment. Its interventions are developmental. It also aligns well with occupational therapy principles being applied to development of aging and aged seniors, facilitated by age-appropriate assessments and interventions.

In some ways, these changes have enlarged the 'therapeutic' role of the activation approach to caring for aging and aged seniors. The activation approach has to a degree enriched the care efforts of social workers and nurses.

Activation programming and programs in long term care is changing. The Age-ability Framework may provide a good way to contextualize the development of activation programming and programs in long term care.

Activation has the potential to bring about creative efforts[35] to generate personal significance, meaning and purpose for aging and aged seniors over and above providing salutary recreation and leisure activities. In this regard, Activation benefits from an Age-ability Framework and can substantially contribute to Age-able programming for aging and aged seniors..

---

[34] Preoccupying an aging and aged woman with a doll will keep her busy and out of trouble, but it is form of restraining development that should be happening to realize the aging and afged woman's present potential.
[35] Such creative efforts are readily recognized in both play and art.

10. Occupational Therapy in Long Term Care: *expanding an established paradigm*

The Canadian Model of Client-Centered Enablement (CMCE) advances 'enablement' as the core competency in Occupational Therapy[36]. In doing so, Occupational Therapy (OT) is transported beyond the limitations of the mechanized biological-medical model approach to human well-being. The leap is further enlarged by *involving meaning as a constituent concern* in the process of a person occupying their existence or existing. Enablement is described as been a) effective, b) minimal, c) missing or d) ineffective.

> *Occupational Therapy is the art and science of enabling engagement in everyday living, through occupation: of enabling people to perform the occupations that foster health and well-being; and of enabling a just and inclusive society so that all people may participate to their potential in the daily occupations of life.*
>
> *Enabling and enablement, focussed on occupation, describe what occupational therapists actually do. Enablement is occupational therapists' core competency.*

The development of an Occupational Therapy program[37] in a long term care home followed the following pathway.

A study of Activities of Daily Living (ADLs) found that these were better described as Behaviours of Daily Living (PBDLs) if the activities were personalized to an actual person and if it was recognized that the personalized activity was functionally dependant on the actual person acting in their actual environment. (Lewin's formula B = P/E.)

*Given a person's past development of critical life skill Preferred Behaviours of Daily Living as integral to their identity, self-concept and esteem, it was observed that aging and aged people have a strong vested preference to perform these critical life skills. The preferential feature was added to aging and aged people's BDLs and called **Preferred Behaviours of Daily Living**. Preferred Behaviours of Daily Living (PBDLs) are Activities of Daily Living (ADLs) considered not simply as abstracted activities, but as actual activities, of a person in their environment, that are vitally important for the person to do. Not performing the PBDL generates stressful anxiety often resulting in maladapted disruptive behaviours. Extending ADLs to PBDLs allows us to utilize an approach that moves from discussing abstractions, to discussion peoples' behaviours in their environments, as a system critical to their survival as a person. Kurt Lewin's formula B <= P/E, can be reworked as follows PBDL <= P/E. Each PBDL is part of an ecological system, whose constituent parts are functionally interdependent.*

It was observed that in the face of changes to PBDLs aging and aged people responded to the changes by overcoming the changes or altering their PBDLs. Some of the changes in their person or in their environment were irreversible. Aging and aged people adapted successfully or maladapted unsuccessfully. It was observed that numerous unsuccessful maladaptations were unacceptably socially

---

[36] Townsend, E.A., & Polatajko, H.J. (2007). *Enabling occupation II: Advancing occupational therapy vision for health, well-being and justice through occupation.* Ottawa, ON: CAOT Publications ACE.

[37] Occupational Therapy For Preferential Behaviours of Daily Living Support Program (unpublished 2014)

and/or were personally disruptive. A program emerged for aging and aged seniors to undo maladapted behaviours and purse successful adaptations in their PBDLs.

Stable PBDL systems are the norm. Destabilized, changed or changing PBDL systems need to be normalized into acceptable risk free behaviours. In particular, those changes in PBDL systems that require normalization and can be normalized in the setting can be dealt by the person through positive behavioural development, with or without support care from caregivers, including support workers, nurses and therapists.

Beside the traditional ADLs, Preferred Behaviour of Daily Living should also include activities such as orientation activity, navigation activity, communication activity, homeostasis activity, self-regulation or self-control (e.g. of anger, frustration, confusion, grief, loss or depression, etc.), and activities of belonging.

We can separate the support provided to residents who's changed Preferred Behaviour of Daily Living can be a) restored, b) restored with a modification in the behaviour, the person or the person's environment (which includes care givers and assistive devices or tools), or c) developed as a new alternate Age-able PBDL. There are other kinds of support (e.g. medication, restraints, etc.) that residents may require due to problematic behaviours.

PBDLs that intimately involved in self-concept, identity and self-esteeming will be done for better or worse by aging seniors. Their sense of personal survival depends on doing them. The done for the better will be successfully adapted; the done for the worse will be maladapted and dysfunctional in one or more ways.

In an effort to ensure they are done for the better, we must take into account the whole PBDL system and its various functionally dependent constituent parts, if we are to properly assess and identify problems with the presenting changed PBDL; and, if we are to identify practical, doable solutions for the presenting changed PBDL problem.

When an intervention targets development of new, alternate PBDL: all the various constituent parts of the PAPBDL system should be considered.

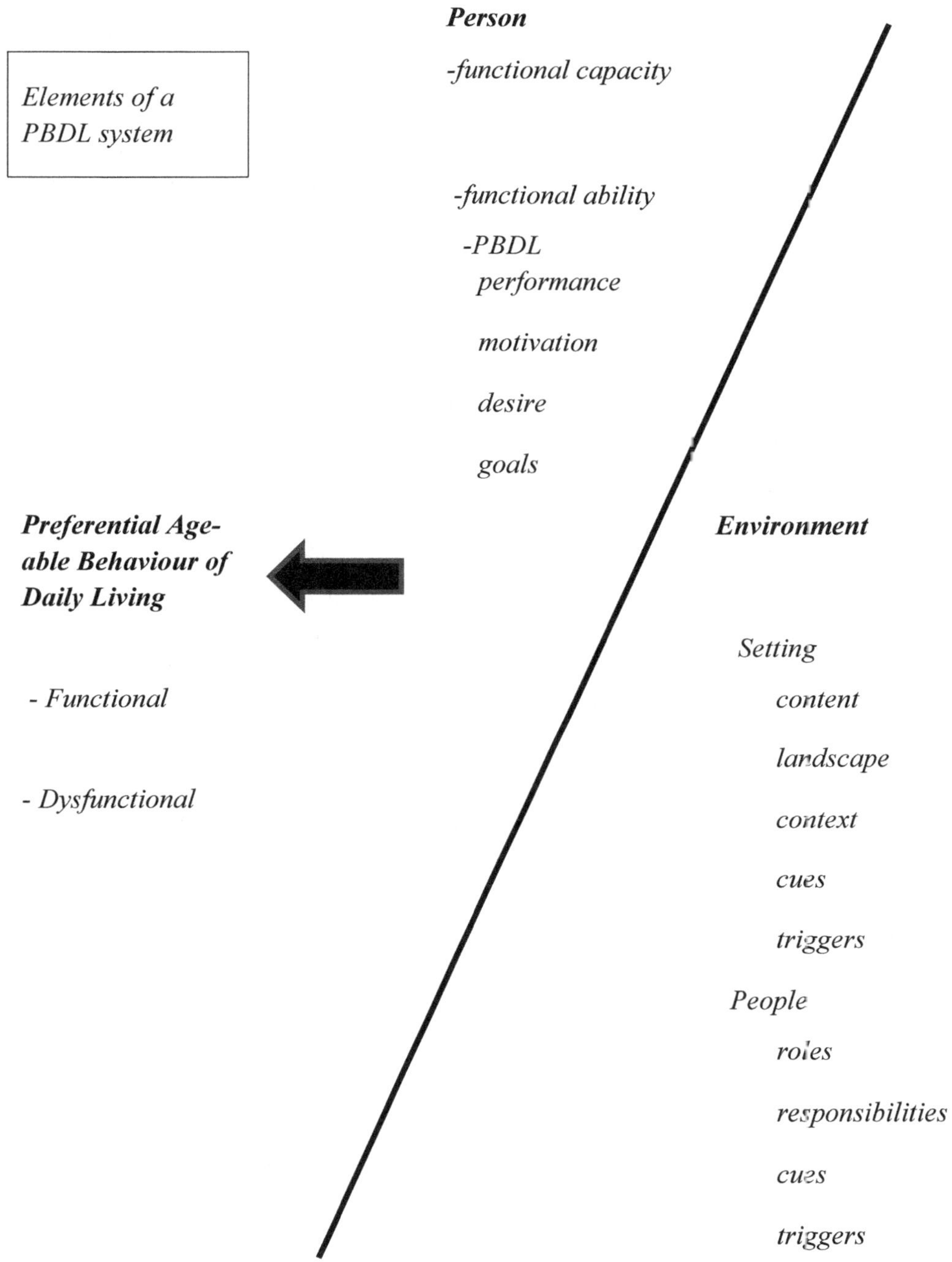

The functional interdependence of the (B <= P/E) formula's various elements and their constituent parts, requires a broad ecological systems approach to supporting changing and changed PBDLs. We can try to identify impending changes and goals to adapt to the changes in order to prepare both the person and the environment (importantly the activities of caregivers) for the imminent challenging changes.

If the PBDL in question is a valued PBDL integrally bound into the person's identity and self-concept, or personal self-esteeming system, it may be driven by one's 'survival instinct'. Old values may need to be released (which is no easy task in the best of circumstances) and new values need to be embraced (which is challenging in the best of circumstances). For example, when independent toileting or transferring is no longer possible, toileting and transferring one's self independently can no longer be and should no longer be valued by either the person or those in his or her environment. Continued valuating of independent self-toileting and self-transferring will drive people who have trouble ambulating and weight bearing to fall or break their bones, and perhaps die. Using a brief and valuing one's intentional competent use of the brief, will allow one to continue with an alternate toileting activity. If valued by the person and those in their environment, the new activity will provide personal satisfaction in toileting by using a brief. Likewise using help of caregivers and lifts for transferring and acquiring the value of one's doable role in the transferring process will facilitate transferring from one position and place to another in a personally satisfying way. This entails changing the parameters and 'norms' of self-actualization. Going from one valued system to the other valued system, involves a lot of change for the PBDL system and all those who are a part of it. Such change involves cognition, emotion, behaviours, social 'norms', cultural ideals, etc.

In searching for a theoretical framework for a PBDL program, it was found that Occupational Therapy's orientation and philosophy is suited to provide a framework for such a program and the Occupation Therapy For Preferred Behaviours of Daily Living was launched in 2014. In retrospect, the program undertakes where possible to do sustainable restoration or rehabilitation of PBDLs. More importantly, in the face of irreversible changes in PBDLs, the occupational therapy program undertakes to do sustainable development of new PBDLs.

*Irreversible changes in critical PBDLs force **a personal paradigm shift** of occupation and occupying activities. The shift may be triggered by cumulative insoluble demands and problems in particular occupying activities. But, it may also be triggered by insoluble demands of the aging and aged person's adult occupation. A new personal occupation must emerge[38], with its own set of critical occupying activities, or critical PBDLs.*

Over time, five basic parts have been identified for the OT PBDL program:

1) *the identification of a particular PBDL that requires support,*

2) *doing a function assessment of the PBDL include scope of sustainable restoration or sustainable development,*

3) *setting restorative or adaptive goal of a. occupational development or b. occupying activity (PBDL) development,*

4) *implementing identified interventions or goal activities to attain goal outcome,*

5) *measuring or evaluating goal outcome.*

Behavioural intentionality comes into play in occupational therapy in a way that it does not in physiotherapy. Why is the person doing an activity helps to determine what the person should be doing, especially if the motivation is to meet a crucial or critical or personal need through development by way personally coping, learning from the coping and then adapting based on the learning from the coping.

---

38 There is a 'model' of such shifting in: T. S. Kuhn, The Structure of Scientific Revolutions, 1st. ed., Chicago: Univ. of Chicago Pr., 1962.

While the occupational therapy profession considers all occupational activities to be occupying activities, there are some activities that are more critical to a person's self-management, self-concept, identity and self-esteem. These *Critical Occupying Activities* (COAs) shape and formulate childhood, adolescent, and adulthood occupations. These critical activities emerge in childhood; develop in adolescence; are performed in adulthood; and morph significantly, based on changing functional capacity, in old age.

When people adapt, their adaptation is either successful or well-adapted to their situation; or alternatively, their adaption is not successful or is mal-adapted to their situation. Mal-adaptions need to be dismantled then reconstructed into successful adaptation of a critical occupying activity or a successful adaption of occupation as a whole. Adaptation is on ongoing response to ongoing changes in critical life skill or COAs. Interventions intended to support successful adaptation requires assessment of the person's functional capacities, as well as assessment as to whether the setting or environment, including caregivers, facilitates or obstructs the performance of the enabled capacity.

Maria Montessori identified critical life skills that children were endeavouring to develop in order to successfully occupy their occupation as children. These Critical Occupying Activities of childhood *purpose learning environments*. Their development are the reasons for preparing learning environments to remove obstacles and facilitate development and mastery of the COAs. Aging and aged seniors for their part also endeavour to master critical occupying activities of their occupation of aging and aged people. Aging and aged seniors undergoing significant change in critical life skills may generate a maladapted, socially disruptive or harmful behavior (activity) of daily living. This maladaptation is driven or purposeful but all the same may not provide the intended goal outcome because it is at odds with their situation.

Childhood, youth and adulthood are well defined occupations that we occupy by developing into them. They are generally recognized and used in the abstract as models of different stages of development. Aging and aged seniors do not have such a well-defined occupation for their stage of development, let alone a developmental pathway leading to such occupation. Each occupation, including that of the aging and aged senior occupation, comes with particular occupying activities. Certain occupying activities like feeding, walking, toileting, transferring, communicating, impulse control or self-management, and reality testing for example, are essential components of personal self-concept, identity and self-esteeming systems of the various stages of life including agedness. Significant irreversible changes due to aging in such 'personally defining' activities or behaviours of daily living that are critical occupying activities, call for significant intervention using occupational therapy.

The role of Occupational Therapy for aging and aged people (including those in long term care) can be enlarged to include articulating the last stage of human life as an occupation with meaningful occupational activities, so as to allow effective enablement for aging and aged seniors to realize successful adaptation based on their current actual functional capacities.

Activation in long term care naturally supports such an inclusion of occupational therapy in long term care. Activation complements the Critical Occupying Activities mentioned above.

The wide spread and enthusiastic use of the Camp's *Montessori Programming for Dementia*[39] (MPD) and Elliot's *Montessori Methods for Dementia*[40] have been well received in recent years, especially in

---

[39] Camp, C.J. (2010), Origins of Montessori Programming for Dementia. Non-Pharmacologic Therapies in Dementia,

dementia care. Some approaches, like Camp's, are an "I am still here." approach. In contrast, Maria Montessori's approach can be considered am "I am going there." approach. Maria Montessori would not favour a 4 year old claiming "I am still here." referring to his or her previous 3 year old self. She would not have set out to sustain the 3 year old self by way rehabilitation or restoration, nor would she be supportive of maintaining the 3 year old person, who has actually become 4 years old. Montessori's observations concluded that children displayed a natural tendency to develop. Children cope with their situations, learn from their coping then adapt. The educator's role was to remove the child's and the child's setting's obstacles and impediments to that natural development. She did make use of sensory and experiential methods to both remove obstacles and impediments from development, and to facilitate opportunities for development. What is true for child development is equally true for aging and aged people's development.

The "I am still here." approach strives to retain the person's past occupation in light of significant changes in critical life skills. Its interventions are rehabilitative, restorative and are at least maintenance oriented. The focus on maintenance can foster a 'dynamic restraining' of aging and aged people by engaging them in and holding them with captivating sensory stimulation and past 'out of context' activities[41], in order to prevent responsive disruptive or harmful behaviours. While it has its use, such dynamic restraining is not the preferred intervention.

The "I am going there." approach strives to support the person's successful coping, learning and adapting of critical life skills based on actual present functional capacities of the person in their setting or environment. Its interventions are developmental. It also aligns well with occupational therapy principles being applied to development of aging and aged seniors, facilitated by age-appropriate assessments and interventions.

It is time to bring the full weight of occupational therapy, including its ergonomics, to bear in creating: tools and instruments suited to aging and aged seniors; as well as purposeful and meaningful activities that are drawn from the richness of the aging and aged stage of life.

People persist in occupying life. Such developmental growth is managed by the person himself or herself; or, it is erratic and responsive to disorganized random events. While occupational therapy supports self-care and self-management, in situations of misfit between real capacity and expectations of capacity, self-management is not viable. At that point, occupational *therapy* involves the birthing of an emergent person. Such occupational *therapy* is not a therapy of correction or rehabilitation. This is particularly true in aging and aged seniors where there is no question of restoring functionality; only the opportunity to develop new functionality based on assessed functional capacities.

In response to irreversible[42] changes due to aging to functional capacities of Critical Occupational Activities (COAs), seniors must transition from one set of functional capacities of activities or preferred

---

[40] Gail M. Elliot, *Montessori Methods for Dementia,* McMaster University, 2011. Elliot seems to go further along the Maria Montessori way.

[41] Preoccupying an aging and aged woman with a doll will keep her busy and out of trouble, but it is form of restraining development that should be happening to realize the aging and afged woman's present potential.

[42] If significant changes to aging are assessed to be reversible, they should be arrested and reverse or restored, treated or cured.

behaviours of everyday living to different sets of everyday living activities or preferred behaviours. Depending of the degree of change, seniors may also have to transition from one occupation (adulthood) to a different occupation (aging or aged senior). Depending on the activities, they may need to transition their identities and all that goes with a person's self-concept, identity and self-esteeming system.

Ineffective enablement attempts to inappropriately encourage, support or to inappropriately undertake to enable performance of activities that a person does not have the functional capacity to do. Whether a person himself or herself undertakes ineffective enablement, or whether caregivers or communities support ineffective enablement, the resources deployed are wasted. The situation is inherently dysfunctional, as well as personally and economically costly. Ineffective enablement is frequently applied in situations where people are unduly attached to maladapted valuations of past activities or occupations, particularly those intimately connected to established self-concepts, identities and self-esteeming systems.

Some aging and aged seniors, their caregivers and communities resist transitioning out of unsustainable adult occupations and states. Some pursue inauthentic mal-adapted transition strategies, which create personal and social dysfunction. This would be ineffective enablement that enables the disruption or dysfunction to persist. In such situations, the solution (i.e. the treatment or cure) may well cause more dysfunction and disruption than the problem (i.e. injury or disease).

As long as aging and aged seniors are bound to previous, now unrealistic occupations, they cannot be free to be what and who they actually are. Properly applied, occupational therapy can engage and enable people to escape from the snares or unreasonable attachments to past functional capacities on which past occupations and occupying activities depended.

The natural and normative process of aging changes more than merely physical capacities. Other capacities are affected, for example cognitive, emotional and accompanying social capacities. The capacity to discern, judge or think critically may change, as might cognitive or behavioural inhibiting. Reality testing, good decision-making and effective problem-solving capacities may change. Such changes in functional capacities will impact on what aging and aged seniors can do and how they do it, as well as on who or what they think they personally are.

If aging and aged seniors are to engage meaningful living and well-being, based on capacities resulting from significant changes due to old age, a lot of developmental work needs to be done by seniors, *as well as* their caregivers and their communities. All this is required at a time when the seniors' critical life skills themselves undergo significant change. Development is most difficult in aging and aged people, and it is most required when they least able to undertake such development.

Occupational Therapy as a discipline has yet to fully include old age in its thinking or to expand its evolving paradigm to embrace aging as a normative development that transitions people from maturity to old age. The Age-ability Framework can be utilized by Occupational Therapy to expand to include aging and aged seniors within their paradigm.

The change from adult to senior, from mature to aged, is not a change due to loss. It is a transition. In occupational therapy (OT) terms, aging should involve a transition of occupation from occupying adult maturity to occupying old age.

When changes due to aging results in loss of mature adult occupation or results in dysfunctional engagement or attachment to an occupation for which there no longer is functional capacity for OT to enable performance, the response(s) may be disruptive to others or to one's self. The disruptiveness would be driven by the strength of person's engagement with their dysfunctional occupation, for example the person's investment in their past no longer valid self-concept or identity. Socially disruptive and harmful behaviours that are intentional can be an effort to deal with or cope with dysfunctional occupation, as best the aging and aged senior can deal or cope with given the capacities and abilities at their disposal.

In order to 'go', aging and aged seniors may need to 'let go' of how they did things and what things they did, in favour of new activities of daily living and new ways of doing the emerging activities of daily living. This applies to the most fundamental activities or preferred behaviours of daily living, as well as the more sophisticated ones. It also applies to occupation as a whole. Seniors whose capacities undergo significant change, need to let go of who they were, in order to successfully be who they are.

In old age, a person's occupation or job is to be aging and aged --- and, a person should be able to do their job well in their *aging and agedness*. To do a god job of being *aged*, a person needs to know what the occupation of being *aged* is and how best to be *aged*.

First, good comprehensive assessments of functional capacities provide the foundation of doing a good job of being aged given the person's functional capacities. Good assessment includes the dynamic at play of performance in a setting or environment, including the role of the person, the environment and their inter-dependence.

Second, the established functional capacities are effectively enabled to develop functional capacities of occupying activities. This is especially needed for the occupying activities that substantively related to and support sustainable personal self-concept, identity and self-esteem.

Third, the person successfully plans to and executes performance of self-managed enabled occupying activities to fulfill their occupational goals and aspirations.

The adult self-managed Activity or Preferred Behaviour of Daily Living **self-toileting** for example, is a complex Critical Occupational Activity that includes the enabled capacity to perform the following tasks:

- transfer to a standing position
- ambulate to the washroom
- transition to sitting
- sit
- urinate or defecate
- clean one-s self
- transfer to standing
- wash hands.

At that point, a person goes away feeling good about themselves.

Sample of successful toileting adapting into agedness.

Constituent Functional Capacities of the toileting COA. (*Other COAs including feeding, ambulating, grooming, etc.*)	**Restorative Therapy** (Physical Therapy to restore capacity and enable physical performance of activity.)	**Adaptive-Restorative Therapy** (Restoring functionality by changing and adapting activity/setting dynamics and tools. Physiotherapy & Occupational Therapy)	**Adaptive Therapy** (Occupational Therapy develops new doable functional COAs and constituent COAs.)
transfer to a standing position	use strengthening and balancing exercises to:	self propel wheelchair into a wheelchair accessible washroom	put on a clean continence product (one piece brief); remove soiled product; self-clean; put on a clean product
ambulate to the washroom	a) remove obstacles or shortfalls to movement;		
transition to sitting	b) restore movement of standing, walking, sitting and hand dexterity.	a. holds onto pull down grab bars to transfer from wheelchair to standing; b. independently unbuckle and doff pants and underwear	
sit		sit	
urinate or defecate		urinate or defecate	
clean one-s self		perform peri-care and don underwear and pants	
transfer to standing		holds onto pull down grab bars to transfer from toilet to wheelchair	
wash hands.		self-propel to sink where its height is appropriate for wheelchair users to independently wash and dry hands	

The adult self-managed Activity or Preferred Behaviour of Daily Living **self-transferring** for example, is a complex COA that includes the enabled capacity to perform the following tasks:

- lift weight off one surface
- bear lifted weight
- reposition body
- release weight bearing
- lower to other surface

Self-managed toileting including transferring are examples of preferred Activities of Daily Living (ADLs) or Preferred Behaviour of Daily Living (PBDLs), which varies from the occupations of a child, an adult and a senior. In all three occupations it is an occupying activity but one that transitions from one set of activities to different sets of activities. Self-managed toileting is also intimately woven into a person's self-concept, identity and self-esteem. Preferred Behaviours of Daily Living that are critical components of an occupation can be referred to as a Critical Occupying Activity (COA). Transitioning from one set of COAs to another involves adaptations to the person's self-concept, identity and self-esteem. Such transitioning calls for unfreezing one occupation's normalized COAs and the formation of a different occupation with new normalized COAs. Other examples of COAs include feeding, walking, self-management, etc.

Toileting, including transferring, is an occupational activity in child, youth, adult and aged occupations. In childhood toileting, including transferring, goes from total dependence to independence, and is supported by parents or caregivers. There some small changes in capacity in toileting, including transferring, in youth; and even fewer in adults. In aging and agedness, changes in capacity become dramatic and significantly impact aging and aged seniors' identity, self-concepts and self-esteeming systems. The changes in functional capacity are extensive and irreversible. In occupying aging and agedness, changes in functional capacity to toilet and transfer are as extreme as or more so than the changes that occurred in childhood. Now, toileting and transferring goes from indepenance to total dependence. This development into aging and agedness may require more adapting than the developments of childhood, and it is required at a time when the aging and aged senior is least able to adapt. The same process applies to all the preferred behaviours of daily living or critical occupying activities.

Charting the COAs orders proper assessment of the functional capacities of occupying activities (for example during times of significant change or during transition, doing assessments quarterly or as required), that then can be organized to enable the therapist to formulate and effectively enable suitable emergent COAs. This is followed by the person and therapist establishing doable self-managed COAs.

Sample of successful transferring adapting into agedness.

Constituent Functional Capacities of the self-transferring COA.	Restorative Assessment and Therapy (Physical Therapy to restore capacity and enable physical performance of activity.)	Adaptive-Restorative Assessment and Therapy (Restoring functionality by changing and adapting activity/setting dynamics and tools. Physiotherapy & Occupational Therapy)	Adaptive Assessment and Therapy (Occupational Therapy develops new doable functional COAs and constituent COAs.)
lift weight off one surface			
bear lifted weight			
reposition body			
release weight bearing			
lower to other surface			

In the face of significant changes in functional capacity due to aging to any or all of those activities, assessments are required to determine new functional capacities and formulate new activities that can be independently performed and self-managed within those new functional capacities, following their effective enablement. Along with assessing the person's functional capacity, the setting or environment (including equipment and people) affects functionality and should also be assessed and altered or adapted. Functional capacity is measured by assessing

1. the individual, [P]
2. the individual's environment(including caregivers and their activities) [E], and
3. the individual performing in the environment. [B]

This transition from one occupying activity to an alternate occupying activity involves a lot of development for successful adaptation. Such intensive and extensive transiting is required on an ongoing basis in all significantly altered COAs, (as well as in other occupying activities) because changes due to aging are ongoing. Below is a suggestive chart comparing transferring as a COA.

The therapeutics of Occupational Therapy in long term care is in construction, not re-construction. The construction uses the person's actual functional assets. The business of Occupational Therapy in long term care is not to make up deficits, but to deploy assets to allow for maximum personal functionality. Occupational Therapy in Long Term Care:

1) assesses to establish the actual present functional capacity of aging and aged seniors in their various settings or environments;
2) effectively enables aging and aged seniors' actual functional capacities; and
3) support aging and aged seniors occupational performance of their occupying activities.

Occupational *Age-Ability* Therapy by Critical Occupying Activity (COA) Capacity Level

Independent/Dependent Co-Functional PABDL Level[43] of Support Care Chart[44]	Long Term Care				
	A	**B**	**C**	**D**	**E**
COA PABDL Enabled Functional Self-Performance	4	3	2	1	0
Supporting Performance Load	0	1	2	3	4
Self-performance Load **Support Worker Load**					
Total	4	2	4	4	4

The goal of Occupational *Age-ability* Therapy is to effectively enable 100% of ***present actual capacity, ability and performance of COA*** *to maximize self-esteeming of oneself in aging and agedness.*

Assessments should reveal:

    a)   what an aging and aged person has the capacity to do,

    b)   to what extent the capacity has been enabled, and

    c)   the aging and aged person's COA self-performance target.

In these notes, there are numerous references to the Gentle Persuasive Approaches training for aging and aged people's care givers. While primarily seen as approach to de-escalate and manage disruptive and increasingly disruptive behaviours, strategies like those utilized in *GPA training can be used to escalate, inflate and encourage positive behaviours. In particular persuasive skills can be applied to escalate the self-performance of Critical Occupying Activities, enhancing positive self-concept, identity and self-esteeming.* Occupational Therapists can use GPA-like and GPA strategies when setting out strategies for care givers to secure aging and aged people's Age-Ability goals.

Strategies like those in the Gentle Persuasive Approaches, can enable and encourage development of *positive Critical Occupying Activities.* When used to escalate or build up behaviours, GPA-like approaches become ability focussed.

---

[43] Level of capacity for self-performance mirrors RAI-MDS measure for self-performance
[44] This chart is drawn from: Di Giovanni, Aldo. *Emergent Seniors' Age-ability Framework: An Ecological Framework for Positively Supporting Preferential Age-able Behaviours of Daily Living*, Charleston, CreateSpace , 2015.

With thorough and detailed assessment by the interdisciplinary team, Occupational Therapists proceed to:

1. Verify actual self-performance Level from A to E. (Aging and aged people should not be admitted to the Occupational Age-ability Program if their score is an E.)
2. Clarify what support workers should do or more importantly should not do. (They should not do what aging and aged people can do; and, should do what aging and aged people cannot do.)
3. Clarify what aging and aged people themselves should do and not do. Undertake to maximize resident occupation (work) within their assessed capacity; minimizing support work as far as possible. Articulate what the resident's 'job' is.
4. Develop an action plan with specific goals to effectively enable abilities, with an outcome of independent self-performance, positively contributing to esteemed self-conceiving, and valued personal identity.
   a. Segment what aging and aged people various performance or learning environment settings
   b. Assess performance setting as a specific learning environment for the particular aging and aged person
   c. Situate active aging and aged people's developmental ability activities in the specific learning environment; accounting for the person and environment functional co-dependence.
   d. Therapeutic activities should
      i. enable the aging and aged person to acquire the ability to self-perform his or her job (occupation) well, and enable the person to actually self-perform their ability successfully
   e. Include measureable outcomes and milestone indicators.
5. Report number of A to D level aging and aged people goals set and achieved.

1. Adaptive-Restorative Program

Ability Level	# Persons	# Goals Set	OT Time	OTA Time	# Goals Done
4					
3					
2					
1					

2. Preferred Behaviours of Daily Living Program

Ability Level	# Persons	# Goals Set	OT Time	OTA Time	# Goals Done
4					
3					
2					
1					

3. Age-Ability Group Program

Ability Level	# Persons	# Goals Set	OT Time	OTA Time	# Goals Done
4					
3					
2					
1					

4. Scanning Learning Environments Program

Ability Level	# Persons	# Goals Set	OT Time	OTA Time	# Goals Done
4					
3					
2					
1					

Summary

Ability Level	# Persons	# Goals Set	OT Time	OTA Time	# Goals Done
4					
3					
2					
1					

11. Social Service Work and Behaviour Care in Long Term Care: *enabling effective enablement*

Changes in fundamental core lifeskills, such as reality testing, inhibiting impulses and delaying gratification, ordering and managing one's self and one's setting or environment as well as the dynamic between the two, call for the kind of therapy provided for within the scope of social service work practice. In the absence of or inadequacy of such fundamental core lifeskills, changes due to aging can trigger maladapted socially disruptive or harmful behaviours, whose management falls within the scope of social service work practice. In either set of circumstances, planning for and implementing successful transitioning fits within the Age-ability Frame for Emergent Seniors.

Social service work assessments and interventions may be word or knowledge based; but they can also be based on interactive and experiential approaches. Changes due to aging (such as those listed above) that affect cognitive and emotional capacities, may be best managed using the interactive or experiential venues to generate insight and establish positive patterns of behaviours, particular behaviours or activities of daily living. What people may reveal what their goal or intention is, and may reveal that the goal and intention has itself become maladapted.

Some social work programs in long term care have been tasked to manage increasing numbers and increasing severities of disruptive behaviours from residents in long term care. This is particularly the case in dealing with intentional but socially disruptive or harmful behaviours that are assessed to not be caused by some physical chemical or pain disturbance. With the advent of the Behaviour Support Ontario program, some social service workers were called on to assume greater participation and leadership roles in the assessment and management of the increasing number and severity of behaviour issues with residents. This was helped by participation in P.I.E.C.E.S. training, which was delivered widely to nurses, especially during the roll out of the Ontario BSO program. This has resulted in a more intensive interdisciplinary approach to managing disruptive behaviour in long term care homes.

Social service work programs (and nursing programs) that emphasized the Capacity part of P.I.E.C.E.S. and looked for interventions suited to the actual presenting capacity of residents, found good resources in the *Gentle Persuasive Approaches, Montessori Program for Dementia* and *Montessori Methods for Dementia* [45]. They gravitated to an asset building or 'abilities' approach to support aging and aged seniors deal with significant changes in their COAs or critical activities of daily living and their response to such changes. The use of Occupational Therapy as outlined in the Occupational Therapy section above would significantly enhance this development.

Transitioning from one positive self-concept to a different and possibly new positive self-concept, from one valued identity to a different or new valued identity, or from one system of self-esteeming to a different or new system of self-esteeming, may require use of diverse and new learning styles by the changed person. For example, aging and aged people may not be amenable to 'talk' therapies or therapies based on verbal instructions; but, they are amenable to

---

[45] See discussion about Montessori in section 9 above.

sensory stimuli or to 'learning' or 'prepared' environments, that facilitate their adapting into their positive development into aging and agedness.

Social service work can enable the effective enablement of actual functional capacities, by other disciplines such as physiotherapy, occupational and activation therapy, as well as its own therapeutic applications.

12. Reframing Nursing Restorative, Behaviour, Dementia and Palliative Care in Long Term Care

In the last 15 years Long Term Care Nursing practice in Ontario has been changing, in particular in regards to restorative, behavioural, dementia and palliative care. In Ontario, the advent of the *2007 Long Term Act and Regulations* and the *Resident Assessment Instrument – Multi-Data Set (RAI-MDS)* brought with them a focus on assessments that emphasized measurement of functional capacity in regards to changing Activities or Behaviours of Daily Living (or what above are called Critical Occupying Activities). Along with those, the use of *P.I.E.C.E.S.*, *Residents' First*, *U-first*, B*ehaviour Support Ontario*, the *Montessori Program for Dementia* and the *Montessori Methods for Dementia*[46] approach, as well as the *Gentle Persuasive Approaches* for staff,   all contributed to an emphasis on measuring functional capacities (including cognitive capacities) in regards to changing Activities or Behaviours of Daily Living and their performance. They also favour selection of care strategies that most supported resident well-being. These trends were supported by the progressions in Activation and Social Work.

The initial nursing response was to enhance nursing restorative care programming with a view to slowing the rate of change of dysfunction, reverse it and cancel out the change by various means. Because changes in functional competence due to aging do not stand still, nursing restorative care responds re-actively. Seniors experience such re-active care as ongoing and persistent loss after loss after loss.

What matters in personal wellbeing of aging and aged seniors is *personally proactive functionality*; not trying to hold on to functionally that is irreversibly changing or changed. Nursing restorative care should be amplified by adding *adaptive care*[47] to restorative care. What emerges is a reframed nursing restorative care that can be called nursing adaptive-restorative care. Nursing adaptive-restorative care proactively approaches changes in seniors' activities or behaviours of daily living that look to assessments of actual functional capacity, then effectively enables that capacity to secure performance that rewards the user with success in achieving *personally attainable and doable goals*.

The attention demanded and the resources utilized in managing the changes and consequences of significant changes resulting in dysfunctional, maladapted and disruptive behaviours in Preferred Behaviours of Daily Living critical to identity, self-concept and esteem, are increasingly consuming nursing time and resources. *Behaviour care focussed on adaptive care should be a 'key result area' in long term care nursing*[48] or, (psychogeriatric nursing aside), in nursing care for aging and aged seniors generally. With the increase socially and personally disruptive as well as harmful behaviours with their attendant problem and risk issues, nursing response in Ontario has been to amplify behaviour care as a care result area for nurses, making liberal use of the *Gentle Persuasive Approaches*, the Montessori Program for Dementia and the *Montessori Methods for Dementia*[49] approach.

---

[46] See discussion about Montessori in section 9 above.

[47] Adaptive care falls under the prevue of Wellness approaches.

[48] Nursing can utilize the approach describe above in the section on Occupational Therapy.

[49] Ibid

Nursing can use the Age-ability Framework to reframe socially and personally disruptive as well as harmful behaviours by considering the intentionality of the behaviour and articulating a nursing behaviour care program that responds to that intentionality. Socially and personally disruptive as well as harmful behaviours may be a mere reflex, for example to pain. But, they may also be maladapted behaviours that are intentionally generated by the person to deal with an issue or problem that is critically important to the person. In the latter case, extinguishing or containing and controlling the behaviour does not address the underlying motivating cause. It will not satisfy the resident's needs. It is the maladaptation that needs to be addressed by putting an successful adaptation in place for the resident. In this regard, nursing can draw on the support of both social service work and occupational therapy to deal with the behavioural and functional dependence between the person and their setting or environment.

Using the P.I.E.C.E.S. assessment tool and the BSO Behaviour Assessment Tool (BAT) with a strong emphasis on functional capacity assessment, helps align nursing behaviour care to the Age-ability Framework. Age-ability Framework interventions can draw in social service, activation and occupational therapy programs to shape a coherent inter-disciplinary response to significant changes and maladapted responses in COAs or activities of daily living that critical to healthy self-concept and personal identity, as well self-esteeming systems.

Disruptive behaviours by aging and aged people have been and are increasingly challenging for care givers to manage and deal with. As a result of such disruption, care giver resources are being unnecessarily consumed when care givers have not been trained to advantageously interact with and de-escalate the disruptions. Extensive training in the Gentle Persuasive Approaches has allowed care givers to more efficiently and effectively manage such disruptive behaviour and avoid their responses to be triggers or accelerators of the disruptions. With the controlling, containment and management of disruptive behaviours, implementation of constructive care plans goes forward according to planned assessments, goals, interventions and evaluations of impact and outcomes.

As mentioned in the section on Occupational Therapy, while primarily seen as approach to de-escalate and manage disruptive and increasingly disruptive behaviours, the strategies in *Gentle Persuasive Approaches (GPA) training can also be used to escalate, inflate and encourage positive behaviours, in particular the Critical Occupying Activities that enhance positive self-concept, identity and self-esteeming*. While GPA effectively helps to contain, control and manage disruptive situations, 'positive' GPA and GPA-like strategies can help staff enable and encourage development. As such, GPA-like strategies can assume a staff abilities approach to caring for aging and aged people.

In 2015, efforts in Ontario Long Term Care Homes to reduce antipsychotic drug interventions without a diagnosis of psychosis, may provide some evidence of the efficacy of a strength based approach to elder care. Some of the residents prescribed antipsychotic drug interventions without a diagnosis of psychosis, were disruptively reacting to significant environmental or personal changes in their lives. They maladapted to the changes. To manage the aggressive and disruptive behaviours medications were utilized. This caused some residents to become slow and drowsy. For a number of reasons, it was determined that use of antipsychotics without a diagnosis of psychosis should be reduced.

Nurses and PSWs, as well as other staff, had in the previous few years been trained in the use Residents' First, the Gentle Persuasive Approaches, Montessori Method for Dementia, P.I.E.C.E.S. assessments and various behaviour support programs. When antipsychotics were being tapered or eliminated, staff applied all their training to:

1) transforming some residents' environments into *learning or prepared* environments and

2) proactively supporting and encouraging residents to, within their abilities, successfully adapt to their situations by coping and developing.

It is also possible that even while medicated, residents were adapting to the changes in environment or personal capacities. The elder care Age-Ability solution is to help residents to successfully adapt by coping within their abilities by adapting themselves or their environments; and, avoid as far as possible the need for chemical interventions.

The *Ontario Long Term Care Act and Regulations*, with its focus on residents' rights and its requirement for a responsive behaviour program created conditions that nurtured the general use of the *Gentle Persuasive Approaches* in staff training to communicate and interact with aging and aged people, and the *Montessori Methods for Dementia* [50] approach to engaging them in activities. These coupled with the various strategies promoted by the Behaviour Support Ontario program, generated a turnaround response to the management of Dementia care in long term care. Containing, controlling and extinguishing so called responsive behaviours, is supplanted by encouraging suitable personally rewarding behaviours in appropriate settings. This approach has been familiar in long term activation programs for many years. It has been adopted in the daily living routines and activities or behaviours of residents that are suited to the functional capacities, abilities and performance.

What holds true for aging and aged people in long term care is also true for aging and aged people at home and in communities.

Another area that has evolved and has generated an emergent abilities approach is palliative care. Palliative care treats aging and aged seniors as they are, providing optimal care given their condition and functionality. With palliative care treatment is redirected, for example from arresting, controlling, or restoring to providing the best care possible to the person as they person actually is. Pain is treated. The person is assessed to determine what they can positively experience as they are and we undertake to support such positive experiencing given what the person can actually do. We alter or adapt the environment the person is in with a view to support positive adaptation to changing conditions. Hubris is set aside. We stop thinking of the person as they were and develop a relationship with them as they are.

Once the decision has been set to participate in palliative care, all care is directed to what the dying person is capable of and helping the person to experience as much as possible with their actual capacities, abilities and performance. Quality of life and living overtakes the forced goal of making up a person's 'deficits' at all costs however diminishing the gain. The trends in conditions that have developed palliative care are similar and have commonalities with what is developing the Age-ability Framework.

---

[50] See discussion about Montessori in section 9 above.

In leading the management of plans of care in long term care, nursing coordinates the integrating and the success of interventions from various disciplines including activation, occupational therapy, social service work and nursing. The disciplines work together utilizing all assessments, all possible interventions and goals and evaluating all outcomes. All the developments in all the disciplines affect the overall care approach.

The ecology of aging and living as an aged senior is shifting towards the development of abilities framework of aging. This is the case in long term care; it is also the case in regards to the provision of care to aging and aged seniors in the community and at home.

13. Seniors Believe Age-ability is Liberating: individual and peer applications of Age-ability in Long Term Care

Given our culture and its history, it is pretty well impossible for anyone to experience healthy aging. Aging demands the most challenging and difficult adaptations and development that we confront in our lives. It takes a life time to prepare for living as an aging and aged senior. Given the amount of change to critical life skills, including cognitive, physical and emotional aspects, can today's aging and aged seniors contribute to their down development into aging and aged senior life? The answer, it seems is yes.

In exploring the Age-ability framework, most seniors (and staff) have positive responses to the approach or culture.

From a long term care residents' council:

- A very large resident's council in a long term care facility adopted the Age-ability approach as their philosophy.

- The residents' council introduces their Age-ability philosophy to newly admitted residents who participate in their meetings.

From a long term care Age-ability peer group:

- A number of residents in a long term care home meet with the home's Occupational Therapist to discuss Age-ability options relating to activities or behaviours of daily living. The residents learn to explore and consider options for changing activities or behaviours of daily living. The OT identifies doable strategies to support group members to achieve their goals.

- As a result of the group meetings numerous referrals were to amending plans of care.

From a senior's personal stories:

- A senior reviewed the Age-ability philosophy then expressed a positive response to what he understood.

- The senior shared the philosophy and its benefits with a committee being interviewed during a long term care home accreditation.

- The same senior was overheard using Skype to share the Age-ability philosophy in his native language with someone overseas.

From a residents' Age-ability Conference:

- Residents in a long term care home prepared for then held an Age-ability 'conference' in which some residents presented the Age-ability approach to the other residents.

- The gathering's theme: how to do a good job of being a senior; or in the phraseology of Occupational Therapy, how to effectively occupy the occupational activities of aging and aged seniors.

From a presentation on Age-ability to a large group of seniors (about 50) in a community seniors' centre:

- Great interest was shown demonstrated by questions during the presentation and after the presentation.

- Numerous seniors approached the presentation to comment and inquire further about application of Age-ability.

- The group want more interaction but time did not allow. They requested a second presentation.

- A few months later a second presentation expanding on the first was presented to about the same number of participants. There were more questions during and after the presentation. They liked the topic and its directions.

9 781974 127818